Demystifying
SYNDROMES

CLINICAL AND EDUCATIONAL
IMPLICATIONS OF COMMON
SYNDROMES ASSOCIATED WITH
PERSONS WITH INTELLECTUAL
DISABILITIES

Editors

Dorothy M. Griffiths

Robert King

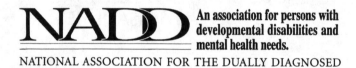

PREFACE

This book was developed to be a practical summary of some of the common syndromes related to developmental disability. The book was designed for:

i.   current professionals working in the field
ii. community college or university students who are studying developmental disabilities
iii. parents, family members, and/or other interested persons who wish to learn more about this area.

The editors have selected some common and some lesser known syndromes that are associated with persons with developmental disabilities and coexisting mental or behavioral challenges, specifically Fragile X, Down, Williams, Smith-Magenis, Pervasive Developmental Disorders, Tourette, 22q Deletion, Smith-Lemli-Opitz, and Angelman Syndrome. Most of the syndromes have known genetic markers for the development of the syndrome. The objective was to demonstrate how and why support and treatment can be individualized by recognizing the differential realities of persons, with various syndromes, who are all labeled as developmentally disabled.

The book was intended to provide a holistic understanding of the biopsychosocial implications of the various syndromes for the lives of persons with developmental disabilities. As such the reader will be provided an integrated understanding of how the physical, psychiatric or biochemical influences may interact with the psychological factors (learning approaches, communication, skills) of the individual, and with the social-environmental aspects (supports, adaptations, and vulnerabilities). The authors have not merely focused on the challenges presented by the syndrome but the strengths and resiliency that each present. Moreover, as much as we have discussed the mental health needs related to the various syndromes, we have attempted to also discuss issues of mental wellness and proactive and preventative intervention strategies.

Simple, non-technical language was used as much as possible. However given the medical complexity of many of the conditions, the appropriate medical terms have been used so that the reader is able to explore these areas further. In some cases, such as chapter 1, a glossary of terms has been included.

CONTENT OF EACH CHAPTER

The chapters have been written by noted professionals working in the field of developmental disability. Although each chapter was written by a different author or group of authors, there was a common outline for each chapter. All the authors were asked to address the syndrome in terms of how it affects the learning and functioning of the person, and what can be done to enhance the functioning and development of the person. Resources have been provided to assist the reader to explore the syndromes further.

This book was not designed to be everything one needs to know about persons with or the genetics of developmental disabilities. The book was developed as a practical guide for current professionals in the field, students in college or university studying developmental disabilities, and parents, family members or other caregivers that wish to learn more about syndromes.

Regardless of the incredible skill that different disciplines bring to the field of developmental disability, this field is rapidly changing and many faceted. As such it is hoped that the book will provide a readable update on some of the research and implications of an area of research and understanding that is literally being uncovered every day. This quote from Dykens, Hodapp, and Finucane (2000, p.21) puts some perspective on this newest shift:

> No one can simultaneously know everything about all aspects of behavior and about all aspects of what is called "the new genetics".... Both personal and disciplinary limits to knowledge suggest caution, even humility.

Chapter 1 provides an introduction to the topic of syndromes and the importance of understanding the influence of syndromes on the biomedical, psychological and social experience of the individual.

Chapters 2-10 provide in-depth descriptions of nine syndromes associated with developmental disabilities and behavioral/emotional challenges. These are Fragile X (Chapter 2), Down syndrome (Chapter 3), Williams syndrome (Chapter 4), Smith-Magenis syndrome (Chapter 5), Pervasive Developmental Disorders (Chapter 6), 22 Q Deletion (Chapter 7), Angelman syndrome (Chapter 8), Tourette's syndrome (Chapter 9), and Smith-Lemli-Opitz syndrome (Chapter 10).

The editors are indebted to the authors who have taken time from their busy clinical practices to share their ideas, insights and research on this important topic.

DEMYSTIFYING SYNDROMES

Editors Dorothy M. Griffiths & Robert King

TABLE OF CONTENTS

CHAPTER 1

Demystifying Syndromes Associated with Developmental Disabilities

Dorothy M. Griffiths & Shelley L. Watson

Why does the man with moderate developmental disability that lives in Welland, Ontario, Canada look, act and talk almost identically to a man in Denver, Colorado, USA?

Why is it that just by looking at some individuals with developmental disabilities that doctors and clinicians can begin to develop theories about their behavior, their medical concerns or their psychiatric states?

Why is it when clinicians hear about certain behavior patterns in persons with developmental disabilities, they start to make associations and begin to ask questions about other behaviors that no one had yet disclosed?

This chapter explores some of the common syndromes associated with intellectual disabilities and the importance of understanding the biopsychosocial implications of the syndromes to support and intervene with individuals with complex needs. The chapter will explore the main reasons to support the identification of syndromes and will use case examples to demonstrate the value of syndromic evaluation.

Introduction

Two young boys were overheard talking at the primary school one day. They were pointing and talking loudly about three boys with special needs. The teacher lingered, curious to know if they were in some way planning to tease or bully these young boys with special needs. (To her delight she found this was her mistaken bias). Instead what the boys were saying was even more amazing to her. They were arguing as to whether the three boys were brothers. The one boy was absolutely sure they were not because they all had different last names, but the other boy was convinced they were brothers because they looked and acted so much alike. By the end they decided they must be cousins, because sometimes cousins look alike. Actually the boys were unrelated at all except through a chromosomal variation that creates Down Syndrome.

Down Syndrome is the one syndrome that most people in the general population can identify. Because it is the most common chromosomal syndrome, the general population has become experienced in identifying individuals who have Down Syndrome. In the mind of the general public, persons with Down Syndrome are for the most part, the typical images of persons with developmental disability. We see people with Down Syndrome as actors on television, models in magazines, and visually portrayed in publicity photos for agencies who serve persons with special needs. See Table 1 for a description of some of the characteristics common to persons with Down Syndrome.

Although Down Syndrome is a common syndrome and many of the associated characteristics of a medical, cognitive or behavioral nature are known to most clinicians and many of the general public, there are many other syndromes that affect developmental functioning that are perhaps not as common or noticeably visible. The general population may not be able to identify the individuals with some of the syndromes as persons with developmental disabilities by sight, but they may know there is something unique about the person. Clinicians too, unless they have experienced many individuals with a particular syndrome, may have difficulty identifying what might be the cause of this person's special cluster of characteristics.

How Syndromes Develop

There is no single gene responsible for intellectual or developmental disability. In fact many causes of intellectual disability have nothing to do with genetics or syndromes. The causes can be the result of prenatal, perinatal or postnatal influences; in other words something that happened before during or after birth. However, research is successfully learning more about the causes of intellectual disability that are related to genetics or specific syndromes.

Genes affect brain development in different ways (how brain is formed in the fetus or in early years, production of brain chemicals or brain regulatory processes) (Dykens et al., 2000). Genes—the factors that determine physical traits—are inherited through chromosomes in the egg and sperm cells (Dykens et al., 2000). Chromosomes contain DNA, which is a "blueprint for how the body develops and functions from conception to death" (Dykens et al., 2000, p. 28). There are 22 pairs of chromosomes

Table 1:

Down Syndrome

Incidence: 1 out of every 700–1,000 live births

Etiology: Extra copy of chromosome 21

How to test: Amniocentesis, chromosome studies

Physical Characteristics

Characteristic facial appearance:

Small head with flat-looking face

Small ears and mouth

Protruding tongue

Upward slant to eyes, with epicanthal folds at inner corners

Broad neck

Short stature

Hypotonia

Increased mobility of joints

Small or undeveloped middle bone of the 5th finger

Single crease across center of palm

Brushfield spots (white spots in iris)

Lack of Moro reflex

Behavioral Characteristics

Often amiable personality, a facility for imitation

Obstinacy, keen sense of the ridiculous, and excellent memory

Alzheimer's disease

15-40% of people with Down syndrome show behavioral symptoms of Alzheimer's, usually after age 45

Depression (please see Chapter 3 for discussion)

Common Medical Vulnerabilities

Congenital heart defects- 50%

Hearing loss (ear infections)- 66-89%

Ophthalmic conditions (strabismus)- 60%

Gastrointestinal- 5%

Hypothyroidism- 50-90%

Dental (crowding, periodontitis)- 60-100%

Orthopedic (atlantoaxial subluxation)- 15%

Obesity- 50-60%

Skin conditions (dry skin, eczema)- 50%

Seizure disorder- 6-13%

Risk of seizures increases with age

Males are generally sterile

Fertility rate in females is low

Women with Down syndrome may be at an increased risk for post-menopausal health disorders, such as breast cancer, depression, and osteoporosis

Alzheimer's disease

After age 30, nearly all people with Down syndrome show the plaques and tangles characteristic of Alzheimer neuropathology, although there is not a direct correlation between plaques and tangles and the severity of Alzheimer's

Preventative strategies
Regular cardiac, hearing, vision, and thyroid exams

Neck radiography after 3 years

Preventative dental care

Weight management

Cognitive Implications

Strengths
Clear developmental trajectory

Visual memory strengths

Sequential processing intact

Can learn sequential tasks well

Weaknesses
Lower IQ scores as develop across childhood/adolescence

Developmental rate slows throughout childhood

Average IQ is 55

Strategies
Manual signs easier to acquire- bridge to verbal language

Acquisition of communication as early as possible

Break tasks into small steps (traditional tasks analysis works well)

Inclusive setting (sociability)

called autosomes and 1 pair of chromosomes that determine gender (XX for female, XY for male). Genes are specific sections on the DNA and there are more than 100,000 genes contained within these chromosomes.

Syndromes can develop in many ways:

♦ *Cytogenetic syndromes* are the result of a difference in the number or structure of the chromosomes (i.e., Down syndrome, Klinefelter syndrome, Turner Syndrome, Cri-du-chat (5p-) syndrome, Smith Magenis syndrome, Prader-Willi syndrome, Angelman syndrome); these typically disrupt many genes and result in a developmental disability.

♦ A single gene causes most genetic conditions (i.e., Smith-Lemli-Opitz syndrome, PKU, Fragile X). Some genetic disorders result from a mutation (nonfamilial) while others are familial and inherited (i.e., Fragile X syndrome).

♦ Patterns of inheritance can occur in three ways:
   i. *dominant inheritance* (where the dominant gene has a 50% chance of being passed from one generation to another),
   ii. *recessive inheritance* (where inheritance is usually within a single generation because it depends on the matching of a recessive gene from both parents), and
   iii. *X-linked inheritance* (where inheritance is linked to a recessive gene on the X or female chromosome); males are always more affected because they have only one X whereas females have a compensating X.

♦ Some disorders are the result of the combined effects of several genes.

♦ Some disorders are the result of a combination of genetic predisposition and environmental factors *(multifactorial)* (i.e., PKU). These disorders cluster in families but are not as predictable as single-gene disorders (Dykens et al., 2000).

♦ The actual cause of some syndromes, such as Tourette's syndrome and Asperger's syndrome, are not yet known, and have yet to be linked to genetic markers.

Until recently the study of genetics was based on examining the inheritance patterns associated with family histories. Many syndromes were identified this way. In the 1960s chromosome studies were able to diagnose some syndromes such as Down and Klinefelter, where the syndrome was caused by an *abnormal number of chromosomes*. However in 1980, Comings discovered that genes could be analyzed at the molecular level, not merely by their consequences (Dykens et al., 2000). High-resolution techniques now make it possible to recognize syndromes that are caused by subtle changes in the chromosomes, such as a deletion or translocations in the chromosome.

Table 2: Types of tests commonly used to determine syndromes

Laboratory Diagnostics	How is it done?	Examples of syndromes that can be so identified
Chromosome studies	Identification of abnormal number of chromosomes through a microscope.	Down syndrome, Klinefelter syndrome
DNA analysis	Presence of gene changes by blood, amniotic fluid, or other body tissues.	Williams syndrome
Linkage analysis	Identifies specific gene change not yet identified by comparing affected and unaffected family members.	Fragile X syndrome
FISH (florescent in situ hybridization)	An artificially created DNA probe with an attached florescent tag, that matches a specific and known chromosome site, can be used to determine the presence or absence of a matching piece of DNA.	Smith-Magenis syndrome

People who work with individuals with developmental disabilities are often amazed at the medical, psychological, social, and behavior complexities presented by individuals with intellectual disabilities. Until recently the complexity of the field was not researched in any systematic way; research was primarily conducted by homogeneously congregating persons with disabilities into one large group. However, in recent years there has been an increased interest in syndrome identification.

The major thrust of this new interest comes from the development of the Human Genome Project. In this project, scientists are uncovering the genetic code of the human body and identifying what genes are responsible for various aspects of human development. They are also identifying how irregularities in genetic development occur, resulting in various syndromes. Today there are known organic causes for approximately 50% of persons with developmental disability (Matalainen, Airaksinen, Mononen, Launiala, & Kaarianinen, 1995; Zigler & Hodapp, 1986); however, not all of these known causes are genetic. Nonetheless, there are approximately 750 different genetic disorders associated with developmental disability (Opitz, 1996). Nevertheless, many of these remain a mystery to professionals working in the field.

Case Example 1

One of the authors was conducting a sexuality consultation recently where a counselor in attendance asked her about a new and unusual case she had just begun. The man, Tim Kingsley, was sticking objects in his orifices (rectum and urethra). This problem had been going on for many years and had been treated in many different ways, most of them punitive and restrictive. The previous agency that served him had assumed that the orifice stuffing was a sexual problem and had treated this by preventing Mr. Kingsley from engaging in this behavior through clothing restraints. He was required to wear jean overalls, secured from being open, all his waking hours. The counselor from the new agency that was supporting him was not comfortable with that approach and wanted to explore alternative options. She was curious as to the motivation or function for this behavior. Was it sexual? Was it a medical problem? She presented this case to the consultant and the consultant started asking questions about Mr. Kingsley.

Q. Does he seem to hug himself (like he is cold)?

R. YES, she said with some reluctance.

Q. Does he put things in his ears or nose?

R. YES AND HE IS ALWAYS PICKING HIS NOSE

Q. Any other self-injury?

R. HE PICKS AT HIS HANDS AND PULLS OUT HIS NAILS

Q. What is his voice like?

R. HOARSE

Q. How does he sleep?

R. VERY POORLY

Q. Does he have vision or hearing problems?

R. YES TO BOTH

Q. Are there any problems with his urinary or fecal incontinence?

R. YES

Q. Do you ever notice there is a problem with his hands and feet?

R. YES HE LIKES TO GET THEM RUBBED AND WILL TRY RUBBING THEM UP AGAINST OTHERS

Q. Does his upper lip look like a cupid's bow?

R. At this point she pulled out a picture of him and said OH MY YES. The woman looked at the consultant and asked "Why these questions?"

The consultant's questions stemmed from associations made with other similar individuals who had been presented with orifice stuffing or digging. They too showed this cluster of behaviors. The consultant's mind wondered back to a brilliant course on Genetics and Developmental Disabilities that she had taken with two of the authors of this book, Brenda Finucane and Elliot Simon, at the International Dual

Diagnosis Certificate Programme in 2001. The consultant wondered "Could it be that this person has Smith-Magenis syndrome? This cluster of behavior and challenges are synchronous to what she remembered about that syndrome." A summary of these characteristics is described in Table 3.

Not being a medical doctor or a geneticist, the consultant suggested that the counselor present this cluster of behaviors, with a copy of a chapter on Smith-Magenis syndrome, to her local physician and seek his advice on whether genetic testing was warranted. He agreed and the family consented.

The counselor had never heard of this syndrome, neither had the general practitioner. That was not surprising because it was not identified until the 1980s and typically goes undiagnosed especially in adults for whom family members have long since stopped asking "Why?"

The Importance of Syndrome Identification

Why is it valuable to identify the syndrome responsible for the disability?

This is a question people often ask when we suggest genetic testing. It is an important question. Persons with developmental disabilities have already been subjected to a host of intelligence and medical tests. Clearly additional testing should have some benefit to the individual if this is to be pursued. Some professionals and family members alike think that genetic testing merely brings a new label to what is already known. They don't feel that a new label can add much to the support or treatment the person may receive; labeling traditionally meant identification of people by intelligence classifications that were not helpful and often harmful. Others argue that so many of the causes of developmental disability are still unknown so there is little to be gained by undergoing testing, which may be time consuming, expensive and inconclusive.

Additionally, some families would prefer not to have genetic testing done. For some families, the idea of genetic testing engenders anticipation of a "cause" that may threaten to create greater guilt or blame than they may be already feeling. For other families, there may be a belief that nothing is to be gained by knowing the cause of their family member's disability. These feelings must of course be respected. Each family must make its own decision regarding genetic or chromosomal testing.

In the above case of Tim Kingsley, both the physician and the counselor asked the consultant a very important question:

"What will this do for Tim if we get a diagnosis of this syndrome?"

Interestingly enough, in his case the family did not ask that question; they still really wanted to know and understand why their son was unique in the manner that he was. They had searched for an answer for so long but had given up. Would this be the answer for them or would it once again be a fruitless effort at understanding Tim's behavior?

Table 3:
Smith-Magenis Syndrome

Incidence: 1 in 25,000

Etiology: Deletion of chromosome 17P11.2 region

How to test: FISH

Physical Characteristics	Behavioral Characteristics	Common Medical Vulnerabilities	Cognitive Implications
Flat mid-face	Do not make any sounds as babies	Some have poor vision (extreme near-sightedness, detached retina)	*Strengths*
Flat head shape	Onychotillomania (picking at/pulling at fingernails and toenails) and polyembolokoilamania (orifice stuffing) are common. In females there may be vaginal stuffing, which may appear like an indicator of sexual abuse, but actually form of self-injury		Long-term memory for places, people, and things
Broad nasal bridge		Hearing impairments	Letter/word recognition
Upper lip shaped like a "cupid's bow"		Sleep abnormalities-aberrant levels of melatonin, leading to disturbed biological clock and circadian rhythm	Simultaneous processing skills
Fair hair and complexion	Self-injurious behaviors- hand biting (most common); head banging (many outgrow this); skin picking		*Weaknesses*
Missing secondary lower bicuspids			Moderate to mild range of intellectual disability
Lurching gait	Sleep disturbances- frequent awakenings at night; deficient REM sleep; early wake-up; narcolepsy-like episodes during day; abnormal melatonin metabolism	Teeth large pulp chambers and low levels of enamel; therefore, get lots of cavities	Weaknesses in sequential processing and visual short-term memory
"stork-like" (thin) appearance to lower legs due to peripheral neuropathy			*Strategies*
	Appreciate attention, and appears to crave one-to-one interactions and may often compete with others for attention; eager to please	Peripheral neuropathy (numbness/tingles in fingers and toes)	Calm, consistent classroom
Dry skin on hand and feet		Scoliosis	Small class size
Short in stature	Perseveration- repeatedly asking the same questions	Chest abnormalities (pes cavus or pes planus)	Reinforcers and motivators
Short fingers	Low impulse control- aggressive hugging, prolonged tantrums, outbursts		
Ear anomalies	Do not adjust well to changes in routine	Chronic ear infections-lead to conductive hearing loss and speech problems	
Deep, hoarse voice	Engaging, endearing, full of personality, a sense of humor		
Strabismus		25% have cardiac problems	
Nearsightedness	Hugging- aggressive (rib-crushing; indiscriminate hugging of others)	Heightened risk of hypothyroidism	
	Self-hugging- almost like a tic "spasmodic upper body squeezing tic thing, with facial grimacing". This is involuntary and appears when excited (less common with age)	Seizures	
		Puberty can be difficult for females;	
	Tactile defensiveness (may present as stripping of clothes)	Urinary tract anomalies	
	Strategies	*Strategies*	
	Care providers need to be: • Emotionally neutral in response to challenges to avoid power struggles • Comfortable with close proximity and have a good sense of humor	Melotonin, in order to reverse melatonin cycle	
	Typically difficult times include transitions from activities and unexpected change; therefore, try to prepare the individual for such changes		

It is important before proceeding with any syndromic testing that a clinician be clear on why s/he wants this syndrome to be identified. Exploring the etiology of a disorder and syndrome identification can be a costly venture, both in time and money. Some physicians may not be as cooperative as Mr. Kingsley's doctor in assisting the process of identification. Some individuals with disability may not want to go through the process or testing. Families may be very reluctant to open this area of pursuit because they either don't want to know or they feel it may lead to disappointment or blame.

There are however some very important and positive benefits of testing for the etiologies of developmental disabilities. Families and service providers should know about the possible benefits so that they can make an informed decision. The authors have identified ten benefits of syndromic identification. These are listed in Table 4.

Table 4: Benefits of Syndromic Identification

1. Syndrome identification helps us understand the reality of the individual.
2. Syndrome identification can lead to increased support for families, caregivers and the individual.
3. Identification of a syndrome can provide invaluable information regarding the individual's learning challenges and may provide collective knowledge that can lead to adaptations.
4. Diagnosis of a syndrome not only allows the challenges presented by the syndrome to be identified, but also the strengths and advantages associated with the syndrome to be recognized and promoted.
5. Many of the syndromes have identifiable strengths which can be developed to promote personal competencies and self-esteem and as compensating features for other challenges. These strengths and approaches can assist in greater learning and less personal frustration.
6. There can be medical prognostic features to the identification of a syndrome.
7. The information can lead to information about mental health risks or resilience of the individual.
8. Identification of a syndrome can lead to communication within clinical and medical disciplines and across disciplines to develop greater understanding and more effective treatment strategies. It may lead to not only clinical and medical collaboration, but to research that can enhance the field and the lives of countless individuals.
9. The nature of the human experience is an interaction of biomedical, psychological and social factors. There are many biopsychosocial implications of identifying the syndromes that individuals possess.
10. Individuals with disabilities or carriers of disabling conditions can gain the knowledge to make informed decisions about reproductive counseling.

Each of these benefits will be elaborated below, using examples of various syndromes to illustrate the points.

First, syndrome identification helps us understand the reality of the individual.

In many situations, knowledge of the syndrome can be very beneficial for the individual's personal plan of support and intervention. Families and caregivers also find that this knowledge brings a renewed understanding of the challenges that the individual experiences and how they can support him/her more effectively.

Understanding the experiences and needs of each unique individual with a disability can be enhanced greatly by knowing the syndrome that caused their disability. With the syndrome identification comes a cluster of cognitive and social strengths and challenges, medical issues, and behaviors. Chromosomal and genetic testing can lead to identification of a syndrome that has a behavioral phenotype or a recognizable pattern of behavior. People who have similar genetic causes of their developmental disability present with similar behavioral phenotypes. A **behavioral phenotype** is a characteristic cluster of behaviors that are associated with a specific syndrome. Some of these phenotypes are unusual and unique to the syndrome. (Dykens et al. 2000) identify as examples, the extreme self injury associated with Lesch-Nyhan syndrome, the high level language abilities coupled with lower overall intelligence level and poor visual spatial functioning associated with Williams syndrome, the hand wringing of Rett syndrome, the cat cry during infants with cri-du-chat syndrome, the self hugging and stuffing of objects into body orifices related to Smith Magenis syndrome, or the food fixation and hyperphagia associated with Prader-Willi syndrome.

Knowing the syndrome can provide important information to the often asked question *"Why do certain individuals behave the way they do and what can be done to assist them?"* The answer is that specific genotypes (e.g., genetic make-up) produce behavioral phenotypes (characteristic behavioral patterns). A definition of a behavioral phenotype is a cluster of motor, cognitive, linguistic and/or social aspects that are associated with a particular biological syndrome (Flint & Yule, 1994). This may also include or may not include psychiatric disorders.

Since the behaviors associated with many syndromes can be very confusing and difficult for families and other care providers or teachers, the identification of the syndrome, coupled with appropriate counseling regarding the syndrome, can be extremely helpful for those supporting the individual. The identification of the behavioral phenotype allows family and others to know what to expect (the trajectory of the syndrome) and how to develop realistic and knowledgeable strategies for supporting the child throughout the lifespan. The behavioral phenotype is not necessarily static; it can change and become more or less prominent at different times through the life. For example the child with autism or Rett syndrome may show no visible signs of a disability until the second year of life. Rett syndrome virtually remains undiagnosed in early years because of the apparent lack of early symptomatology. However, once skill deterioration begins, families become frantic to search for an explanation for the devastating change in their child's development. (See Table 5 for a description of Rett syndrome).

Table 5:

Rett's Syndrome

Incidence: Primarily in females

1 in 10,000 female births

Etiology: Mutations in the MECP2 gene on the X chromosome

How to test: Molecular analysis of the MECP2 gene

Physical Characteristics	Behavioral Characteristics	Common Medical Vulnerabilities	Cognitive Implications
Wide-based gait, similar to Angelman syndrome	Period of regression, withdrawal (normal progress from 6 to 18 months)	Seizures	*Strength* Very expressive eyes
Poor circulation- cold hands and feet		Hyperventilation	*Weaknesses* Severe to profound intellectual disability
High metabolic rate	Loss of acquired hand and speech skills by age 1-2 years	Central breathing dysfunction	
Scoliosis		Sleep disturbance- 70%	Severe, impaired expressive and receptive language develop between 1-4 years
Very expressive eyes	Onset of stereotypies- hand wringing or washing, hand mouthing	Scoliosis	
Normal head size at birth, but slowed growth between 5 months and 4 years		Constipation	*Strategies* Communication board
	Lifelong stereotypies- often unable to use hands	*Strategies* Pharmacological, especially for seizures	
Hypotrophic (underdeveloped) small feet	Self-injury- 40-50%	Careful monitoring of scoliosis	

Second, syndrome identification can lead to increased support for families, caregivers, and the individual.

Identification of the syndrome that created the specific behavioral phenotype in the individual can also be extremely helpful for families at many levels. First, there is the obvious understanding that can come with the knowledge of how their family member came to have their unique special need and how the syndrome relates to the biological, social and psychological profile the person presents.

Second, families often experience considerable guilt or self-doubt that they may have done something wrong to cause the disability. Understanding the nature of the development of a syndrome can in many ways relieve that guilt. One of the authors remembers one mother saying, " So it was not that glass of wine I had at my cousin's wedding that caused Johnny to have a developmental disability". She was so relieved to know that she was not responsible by her actions for her son's challenges.

Third, and perhaps the most valuable reason for appropriate diagnosis for a family, is the opportunity that identification provides to connect this family with other families who have a member with the same syndrome. With the invention of the Internet, families all over the world can easily share stories, information, strategies, and supports with each other. This type of support can be especially invaluable for families with young children who are learning about the complexity of their family member. Similarly, teachers and care providers can share information that can enhance their interactions with the child. Likewise, of special benefit is that the individuals themselves often enjoy being part of an identifiable peer group. It is very heartening for individuals with Williams syndrome to be able to get together and share their stories of their unique talents, to hear individual's with Tourette's syndrome speak as a group with pride about their special gifts, or to see the joy when a group of persons with Down syndrome note that they think they should rename their syndrome to Up syndrome because there is nothing negative about them.

Third, identification of a syndrome can provide invaluable information regarding the individual's unique learning challenges that may provide collective knowledge that can lead to adaptations.

Case Example 2

Roger LaPierre was referred for an assessment following his placement in a new integrated work program that was associated with a large factory. Mr. LaPierre and seven of his colleagues worked in an enclave of a large factory. He has excellent long-term memory and good expressive and receptive verbal language relative to his overall abilities, but he appeared to be extremely shy and anxious. The staff member that operated the program thought he would do well in an integrated setting. His job consisted of working on an assembly line. He and the individual across from him on the line would be working together on their piece of the assembly. The assembly task involved rotating and attaching several pieces to make a whole. The task consisted of a moderate degree of sustained attention. The staff member knew that some people had problems with the task and so she explained the job to him several times. She felt confident that he would be able to do the task because of his good verbal skills; he was able to repeat the instruction phrases. However, an hour or so following the training session he became very aroused and anxious. He seemed anxious and aroused during the training. It appeared as if the noise from the factory was causing him some discomfort but he did not react immediately. However, about an hour after the training session he began to bite his wrists to the point where he drew blood. When the staff member intervened to try to get him to attend and look at her so she could discuss his distress, he became verbally aggressive. The staff was stunned. What brought this on? They looked at the environment and could not see what triggered this behavior.

Many individuals with intellectual disabilities would have coped well with this setting. It was highly structured and the assembly task was one that other persons in the program had mastered easily with instruction. However for Mr. LaPierre, this environment was a culmination of a variety of environmental and social triggers that he was particularly vulnerable to because of the nature of his syndrome. Mr. LaPierre had Fragile X syndrome.

In examining Table 6 it can be seen how the environment in which he was placed was a critical influence on triggering this behavioral event. First, the environment was noisy and over-stimulating. Second, the nature of the task required that he a) sit across from another individual, hence forcing eye contact, which for him is very aversive, and b) use both sequential processing skills (following several steps) as well as visual spatial perceptual organizing skills (rotating the object). These are both challenges for him. Third, the instructor's method of teaching was based on auditory verbal instruction, rather than imitation. Fourth, the instructor's efforts at intervention once he was over-aroused, was to require him to look at her so she could calm him down; in his case, his aversion for eye contact would result in the opposite effect that she desired.

Table 6:

Fragile X Syndrome

Incidence: 1 in 1,500 males and 1 in 2,500 females

Most common hereditary cause of intellectual disabilities in all populations

Etiology: Unusual X-linked pattern related to trinucleotide repeat expansion

How to test: Analysis

Physical Characteristics	Behavioral Characteristics	Common Medical Vulnerabilities	Cognitive Implications
Macrocephaly	Speech pattern- short bursts, repeat phrases	Mitral valve prolapse- only significant medical issue	*Strengths*
Large ears	Imitation skills with inflection	Seizures- 20%	Excellent long-term memory
Long, narrow face	Delayed emotional reactions	Strabismus	Verbal skills
Macroorchidism	Stalling- avoidance	Scoliosis	Repertoire of acquired knowledge
Low muscle tone	Overreaction to minor events	Sinus problems	Expressive and receptive vocabularies
Hyperextensible joints	Attention deficits	Atlantoaxial dislocation	*Weaknesses*
Flat feet	Verbal vs. physical aggression		Auditory-verbal short-term memory
Soft skin	Gaze aversion (not just poor eye contact)- starts at age 2		Visual-perceptual short-term memory
	Hyperarousal is often the root of anxiety (eye contact, overstimulation); this is demonstrated by self-injury (hand, wrist-biting); mouthing objects and clothes; hand flapping		Sequential processing
	Strategies		Sustaining attention
	Be aware of anxiety triggers:		Integrating information
	Forced eye contact		Certain visual-spatial and perceptual organization tasks
	Personal space		*Strategies*
	Tactile defensiveness		Teach task to another student; child with Fragile X will observe and learn task
	Emotional tone of peers and staff		Respond well to structure and routine
	Changes in routine		
	Auditory stimuli		
	Changes in environment		

If the instructor had known about Mr. LaPierre's syndrome and what his sensitivities and challenges were, this situation need not have occurred. So often persons with intellectual disabilities experience this type of disharmony in their programming and are often "blamed" for the failure. In reality, it is an inappropriate matching that resulted from a lack of knowledge about the individuals that are being supported; syndromic identification provides many pieces of that knowledge base necessary for setting people up for experiencing success not failure.

Fourth, diagnosis of a syndrome not only allows the challenges presented by the syndrome to be identified, but also the strengths and advantages associated with the syndrome to be recognized and promoted.

Case Example 3

At a recent plenary session at the annual conference of NADD (Association that serves persons with mental health needs and developmental disabilities-dual diagnosis), a woman was introduced by her father to the hundreds of conference attendees. She took the stage and began to sing a series of songs in perfect pitch. She sang both classical and popular music with equal ease. Her presentation was confident; she was comfortable in this public appearance, and tremendously talented. What might have been surprising to many was that this woman had Williams syndrome and had an intellectual disability.

We often think of persons with intellectual disabilities as a compilation of challenges and deficits. Yet many of the syndromes also present with skill and ability strengths and in some cases remarkable abilities. Persons with Williams syndrome provide a perfect example of these strengths (See Table 7). Their sociability and musical talents are amazing and can be developed to provide the individual with enormous pleasure and development. Similarly, persons with Tourette syndrome present with both strengths and challenges associated with the syndrome. (see Table 8)

So often when we think of a person having a syndrome related to a developmental disability we think of the limitations or challenges that the syndrome may present for the person. However, so many of the syndromes also have associated strengths that are overlooked. These strengths can serve as resiliency factors for the mental wellbeing of the individual and may enable the person to live a more positive life. The individual may demonstrate skills, talents or abilities that distinguish him or her with areas of strength, that if capitalized on by the individual, can bring great satisfaction and achievement, as in the case above.

Whether we are talking about the:

♦ perfect musical pitch, sociability and kind spirit of persons with Williams syndrome,
♦ mental health resilience and adaptive daily functioning and social skills of persons with Down Syndrome,
♦ strong verbal skills, long- term memory abilities, and daily living skills of persons with Fragile X syndrome,
♦ energy, sociability and helping nature of persons with Prader-Willi syndrome,

- happy personality of persons with Angelman's syndrome, or
- exceptional organizational skills and creativity of persons with Tourette's syndrome,

it is evident that syndromes not only come with some challenges but strengths that can be used in educational and social settings to maximize a person's potential for happiness and success.

Table 7:

Williams Syndrome

Incidence: 1 in 20,000 live births

Etiology: Contiguous deletion of area on chromosome 7

How to test: FISH test

Physical Characteristics	Behavioral Characteristics	Common Medical Vulnerabilities	Cognitive Implications
Characteristic face:	Sociability	Infantile hypercalcemia	*Strengths*
Elfin-like appearance	High rates of anxiety/fears/phobias	Supravalvular aortic sclerosis- at least 75%	Verbal abilities and expressive language
Short, upturned nose	Friendly demeanor- no stranger anxiety	Other cardiac problems	Facial recognition
Long philtrum		Hypertension	Musical talents
Broad forehead with bitemporal narrowing	95%- Hyperacusis/hypersensitivity to sound- increased startle response (cover ears)	Peptic ulcers, diverticulitis	*Weaknesses* Mild to moderate ID
Full cheeks		Constipation, abdominal pain	Major impairments in visual spatial tasks
Puffiness under the eyes		Otitis Media	
Prominent earlobes	Musical talents- increased interest in music; perfect pitch	Premature aging of the skin	*Strategies* Talk through problems- verbal mediation
70% have starburst pattern in iris	Difficulty making or keeping friends	Tendency to develop hernias, urinary tract infections, and bladder diverticulae	Learning to read- letter/sound associations
Hoarse voice	Vulnerable to exploitation		Learning to write- raised line paper
Hyperextensible joints	*Strategies* Music therapy or lessons	Strabismus	
	Minimize distractions (Ritalin)	Atlantoaxial dislocation	
	Sound sensitivity management	*Strategies* Low calcium diet	
	Be attuned to obsessions- set boundaries	Cardiologist	
	Social skills training		
	Anxiety/phobia management		
	Comfort/reassure/move on		
	Cognitive behavior therapy- systematic desensitization		
	Attune to underlying sadness/depression		

Table 8:
Tourette's Syndrome

Incidence: Males: 1-8 in 1,000 live births
               Females: 0.1-4 in 1,000 live births

Etiology: UNKNOWN

How to test: See DSM-IV criteria

Physical Characteristics	Behavioral Characteristics	Common Medical Vulnerabilities	Cognitive Implications
No specific physical characteristics	Symptoms begin between the ages of 2 and 15 years, but most people have symptoms by age 11	Sleep disorders are common	*Strengths* Organized way of thinking
	Hyperactivity and impulsivity are common	No specific medical issues, although suppression of tics may lead to injury when they are finally released	Creativity
	Complex motor and vocal tics occur in varying combinations and that wax and wane		*Weaknesses* Delays in speech development
	Motor tics (simple): Abdominal tensing, arm, hand, or head jerking, echokinesis, finger movements, facial movements, rapid kicks, shoulder shrugs, bruxism.	*Strategies* Pharmacological management with drugs such as SSRIs, adrenergic agonists, dopamine antagonists, calcium channel blockers, and atypical anti-psychotics	20% prevalence of math and written language disabilities
	Motor tics (complex): Adjusting clothing, arranging things, biting, body rocking, clapping, copropraxia, echopraxia, head banging, hitting, hopping/jumping/skipping, kissing, picking, sniffing/smelling, touching genitals (self or others), writing same word over and over		Visual motor deficits on copying tasks
	Vocal tics (simple): Barking, belching, blowing, chewing, coughing, grunting, screeching, shrieking, snorting, whistling		Fine motor skill deficits (i.e., poor handwriting)
	Vocal tics (complex): Coprolalia (in only 20% or so), counting rituals, echolalia, insults, laughing, mental coprolalia, partial words, stammering or stuttering, stereotyped expressions		*Strategies* Create a quiet, separate space for test completion
	Strategies Perhaps tic reduction should not be the goal, rather awareness of the context in which tics are occurring as well as factors that increase impulse to tic		Testing with modalities other than timed written examinations
	Suppression of tics can lead to lowered self-esteem and depression		Assigning tasks one by one, rather than as a sequence
	Unrestriction/ encouragement of minor tics		
	Development of "Tourette's Pride" and preserving and fostering self-esteem ("It's OK to tic")		
	Education to clients, families, and caregivers		
	Expression through exercise, dance or music		
	Visiting places where tics are not as noticeable (i.e., baseball games)		
	Pharmacotherapy		

Fifth, many of the syndromes have identifiable strengths which can be developed to promote personal competencies and self-esteem and as compensating features for other challenges. These strengths and approaches can assist in greater learning and less personal frustration.

Intervention strategies were historically reactive, meaning that individuals were provided appropriate intervention, if and only if they presented with challenges. The reactive strategies were typically of a punitive or aversive nature. However, in recent decades there has been a movement in the field towards strategies that are more proactive, preventative, and positive supports and interventions. Understanding the challenges and strengths that an individual has can lead to the development of a support and intervention plan that is positive and preventative.

POSITIVE support and intervention for persons with a developmental or intellectual disability refers to:

♦ the addition of events, reinforcements, activities to the environment and interactions
♦ promotion of the development and maintenance of functional behavior serving to bring the individual natural positive rewards and
♦ allowing the individual to escape from and avoid situations that bring internal distress and discomfort (Griffiths, Gardner, & Nugent, 1998).

By understanding the nature of the syndrome, it is more likely that environments and interactions can be developed that will bring the individual greater natural rewards and avoid situations that may predictably bring distress.

Just as different individuals in the general population may learn best using different approaches and modalities, research has shown that persons who experience different syndromes have identifiable ways in which their learning can be enhanced.

Oliver Sacks, in his amazing book *An Anthropologist on Mars* (1995) cites a quote from L. S. Vygotsky, one of the classic learning theorists, who suggested many years ago that:

> *A handicapped child represents a qualitatively different, unique type of development…[if a child with a disability] achieves the same level of development as a normal child, then the child…achieves this in another way, by another course, by other means; and for the pedagogue, it is particularly important to know the uniqueness of the course along which he must lead the child. This uniqueness transforms the minus of the handicap into the plus of compensation (xvii).*

Research has shown:

♦ Persons with Williams syndrome have great verbal expressive skills and great strength in facial recognition.
♦ Persons with Angelman syndrome demonstrate strength in receptive language.

- Long-term memory for places, people, and things, letter/word recognition, simultaneous processing skills, expressive language development higher than would be predicted based on overall level of cognitive functioning in persons with Smith-Magenis syndrome.
- Persons with Down syndrome have particular visual memory strengths and abilities in sequential processing and tasks.
- Excellent long-term memory, verbal skills, a repertoire of acquired knowledge, and expressive and receptive vocabularies are strengths of persons with Fragile X syndrome (Dykens et al., 2000).

All of these strengths are the unique paths by which the disability can be transformed, as Vygotsky (1993) suggests, into a very positive compensation strategy. Rather than focusing on the aspects of life that the person may not be able to achieve or may not wish to explore, enhance and explore those areas where the person gains pleasure and derives success.

The brain is remarkably adaptive to the needs of the individual and the unique diversity of the brain development (Luria, 1966). Clinicians who understand the learning strengths and challenges of an individual can develop strategies to allow for adaptations. People do not all learn in the same manner. Some people learn best through audio (hearing), some through visual (seeing), and others need things modeled for them. The brain is remarkably adaptable and creates new organization and order to allow the person to compensate; however learning strategies need to be developed to ensure that the individual is able to learn in the best modality that suits their learning style.

Some specific learning strategies are follows:

- For individuals with Fragile X syndrome, de-emphasis on auditory short-term memory and emphasis on visual integration and contextual learning is important (Dykens & Hodapp, 1997).
- For individuals with Williams syndrome, written tasks should be de-emphasized; strategies such as computers, calculators are recommended (Dykens & Hodapp, 1997).

Sixth, there can be medical prognostic features to the identification of a syndrome.

Knowledge of the potential medical risks associated with the syndrome can provide direction for care providers and medical personnel to a proactive program of medical care. Additionally, the information provides direction for intervention related to some associated challenges.

In general:

> Because of Mr. Kingsley's syndrome, he should have regular hearing, dental and vision checks (near-sightedness and risk of detached retina). There should be increased medical awareness risk of cardiac problems, hypothyroidism, chest abnormalities, scoliosis, seizures, and chronic ear infections.

> However specific to his presenting challenges we can also learn some valuable information: Mr. Kingsley was noted for "frottage"(rubbing himself up against others). Reports in his file showed that this had been considered a problem in the past because he would always try to rub his feet up against staff and other residents. He had been on several behavioral programs to stop this behavior but the effects were always short lived. Knowledge that Mr. Kingsley had Smith Magenis syndrome and probably was experiencing peripheral neuropathy (numbness and tingling in the fingers and toes) provided valuable information that would produce both a more effective program and also one which took into account the distress he was experiencing. In this case, it was suggested that his hands and feet be massaged regularly with medicinal cream that would ease the tingling. Mr. Kingsley was taught how to ask for this therapy whenever he felt the discomfort. He was also taught how to do this himself.

In general, research has shown that different syndromes are associated with potential medical challenges and risks. By knowing these potential risks, physicians can be routinely testing for high-risk medical situations that are associated with these conditions and perform preventative and proactive medical care.

One of the most remarkable outcomes from identification of a genetic condition is phenylketonuria, often called PKU. Developmental disability is caused when these children fail to metabolize the amino acid phenylalanine. However diagnosis followed by a specialized diet can alleviate the effects of the genetic disorder leaving only subtle cognitive and attention problems, where otherwise severe/profound developmental challenges would have occurred (Dykens et al., 2000).

Knowledge of the nature and trajectory of the syndrome allows care providers to be *PROACTIVE* in their approach. Medical challenges are commonly associated with various syndromes, for example,

♦ persons with Angelman, Rett, Fragile X and Smith Magenis syndrome are more susceptible to scoliosis,
♦ persons with Down syndrome, Smith Magenis, Smith-Lemli-Opitz and 22 Q Deletion syndrome often experience heart defects,
♦ sleep disorders are common in persons with Rett, Tourette's, Angelman, and Smith- Magenis syndrome, and in the latter case, melatonin has been shown to be of great value in many individuals,
♦ persons with Smith Magenis syndrome have heightened risk of hypothyroidism, ear infections, and experience peripheral neuropathy,
♦ seizures are more likely in persons with Rett, Smith-Magenis, Fragile X syndrome,
♦ persons with Fragile X may experience mitral valve prolapse,
♦ women with Down syndrome may be at greater risk of post menopausal heath disorders such as osteoporosis and breast cancer,
♦ Hirschsprung's disease is common in Smith-Lemli-Opitz syndrome, and
♦ hearing loss is common in persons with Smith-Lemli-Opitz, Down, and Smith-Magenis syndrome. (See more on Smith-Lemli-Opitz syndrome in Table 9)

19

Table 9:

Smith-Lemli-Opitz Syndrome

Incidence: 1 in 40,000 live births

Etiology: Autosomal recessive disorder of cholesterol metabolism

How to test: 7 dehydrocholesterol analysis

Physical Characteristics	Behavioral Characteristics	Common Medical Vulnerabilities	Cognitive Implications
Epicanthal folds	Feeding problems as babies	Low blood cholesterol level	*Strengths*
Ptosis	Behavioral difficulties or autistic features	Cataracts	Acquisition of good language and adaptive skills is common
Microcephaly		Cardiac defect	
Small jaw		Liver disease	*Weaknesses*
Small upturned nose		Hirschsprung's disease (absent nerves in colon)	Intellectual disability
2nd and 3rd toe syndachtyly (95%)		Constipation	Expressive language disorder
Short thumbs		Hearing loss is common	*Strategies*
Postaxial polydactyly		*Strategies*	Speech therapy
Cleft palate		Dietary therapy, aimed at correcting cholesterol deficiency	Audiology
Hypotonia		Rectal biopsy may be useful when Hirschsprung disease is suspected	
Genital malformations from hypospadias to female genitalia in boys		Hearing tests are important due to risk of hearing loss	

Seventh, the information can lead to information about mental health risks or resilience of the individual.

Here are a few examples:

♦ Persons with Down syndrome appear to have lower levels of psychopathology (Hodapp, 1997); however, postmenopausal females are more susceptible to depression.

♦ Persons with Fragile X often experience anxiety disorder that is responsive to medications and environmental changes.

♦ Individuals with Prader-Willi syndrome often experience mood swings that are aided with medication.

♦ Persons with Smith-Magenis syndrome often experience severe sleep disorders.

♦ Caution needs to be used with persons with Angelman syndrome because their behavioral characteristics (hyperactivity, frequent smiling and laughter, sleep disorders) often lead to a misdiagnosis of bipolar disorder.

♦ Persons with 22q Deletion Syndrome (Table 9 below) are often diagnosed with ADHD, Impulse control disorder, Obsessive Compulsive Disorder, anxiety disorder, and Depression (facial hypotonia) during school age. Later, 29% meet criteria for schizophrenia/schizo-affective disorder (Pulver et al., 1994) and 64% meet criteria for bipolar spectrum disorder (Papolos et al., 1998). (See more on 22q Deletion Syndrome in Table 10).

Table 10:

22q Deletion Syndrome

Formerly known as DiGeorge syndrome, conotruncal anomaly face (CTAF) syndrome, Velocardiofacial syndrome, Shprintzen syndrome

Incidence: 1 in 4,000 live births

Etiology: Microdeletion on the long arm of chromosome 22

How to test: FISH test

Physical Characteristics	Behavioral Characteristics	Common Medical Vulnerabilities	Cognitive Implications
Characteristic facial appearance:	Hypernasal voice	Highly variable congenital anomaly syndrome (different organs affected)	*Strengths* Verbal IQ
Flat affect (often hard to see)	At school age, often diagnosed with ADD, impulse control disorder, OCD, anxiety disorder	Congenital heart defects- 80% born with cardiac defects ranging from minor to severe	Verbal processing
Long, featureless philtrum			Rote verbal learning and rote verbal memory
Thin upper lip	Depression (facial hypotonia)		Initial auditory attention and simple focused attention
Small mouth	In adolescence, 29% meet criteria for schizophrenia/ schizo-affective disorder (Pulver et al., 1994) and 64% meet criteria for bipolar spectrum disorder (Papolos et al., 1998)	- tetralogy of fallot	Auditory perception and memory
Prominent nasal root		- interrupted aortic arch	
Large nose with large tip		- truncus arteriosus	Word reading and word decoding
Narrow, "squinting" eyes		- VSD	
Small ears with thick, overfolded helixes		Immune deficiency	*Weaknesses* Common cause of learning disability and intellectual disability
Oral clefts		Feeding/swallowing problems	Non-verbal processing
		Hypocalcemia	Visual-spatial skills
		Growth hormone deficiency	Complex verbal memory
			Facial processing and recall
			Phonological processing
			Deficits in language processing
			Mathematics and reading comprehension

These potential protective features and vulnerabilities or risk factors can be important to know. They can assist in appropriate diagnosis and treatment of identifiable conditions that have a known path of intervention. This knowledge can also assist in appropriate differential diagnosis (i.e., identifying what is really going on and eliminating possible rival hypotheses that wold lead to a misdiagnosis).

Eighth, the nature of the human experience is an interaction of biomedical, psychological, and social factors. There are many biopsychosocial implications of identifying the syndromes that individuals possess.

An integrative biopsychosocial model is based on the premise that behavioural and emotional challenges faced by persons with developmental disabilities represents the *dynamic* influence of biomedical, including psychiatric and neuropsychiatric, psychological and social environmental factors (Griffiths et al., 1998; Griffiths & Gardner, 2002). Each factor may play not only an individual role in the expression of symptoms, but factors may interplay to influence features of the behavioral challenges.

Using this model, the challenging behaviour, rather than being the focus of assessment and intervention, is viewed as a symptom of other conditions. In viewing behavioral challenges as a symptom, the diagnostic and intervention attention is immediately shifted from the behavior to those conditions that produce the behavioral symptom. The behavior itself tells us nothing about the controlling conditions that influence its occurrence, severity, variability, or durability. Aggression, for example, may be influenced by medical, psychiatric, and neuropsychiatric influences, social interactions, physical and program environmental events, psychological needs or distress, or may reflect the absence of alternative ways to deal with any of the above. Thus, reduction or elimination of the behavioural challenge is not the goal of the clinical approach. Rather, identification and modification of the various conditions (causes) do represent the focus. For an example of the application of this model to a case of Fragile X refer to (Griffiths & Gardner 2002).

So back to Tim Kingsley: Why did we want Tim to be tested for Smith-Magenis syndrome?

Case Example 1 Revisited

Tim Kingsley was experiencing a very restricted lifestyle because of his behavior challenges and the fact that individuals who were supporting him did not have the understanding regarding the nature of his behavior to assist him. He was in clothing restraints (overalls zipped at the back) and was being denied time to engage in sexual satisfaction because of fear of injury. He had been on many highly intrusive behavioral programs to attempt to modify his self-injurious behavior, but without success.

Moreover, he was causing considerable disruption in his home due to his sleeping problems. He was rarely taken into the community because of his behaviors and he spent much of his time in isolated activities. This was problematic for Mr. Kingsley as he very much enjoyed individual attention and demonstrated a great need to please others. He was however continually disappointing his family because of his perseverative behavior.

By knowing that Tim may have Smith-Magenis syndrome, several things might change:

First, the people that support him would understand that there was some internal reason that was causing his self-injury. Individuals with Smith-Magenis syndrome become more agitated if physically restrained from engaging in this behavior. Thus, instead of punishment and restraint, creative options to alter the internal sensations that were causing the self-injury would be more likely to be entertained (i.e., use of creams or massage machines to stimulate his peripheral neuropathy).

Second, research has shown that there may be some medications (i.e., melatonin) that have been shown to be effective with persons with Smith-Magenis syndrome to regulate sleep.

Third, the strengths associated with Smith-Magenis syndrome could be optimized. Although it was true that he had problems in visual short-term memory and sequential processing, Tim had an excellent long-term memory for places, people and things. He was good at letter/word recognition and had simultaneous processing skills. He also had expressive skills that were higher than predicted by his overall cognitive functioning. His environment could be adapted to minimize reliance on areas where he had challenges and maximize his strengths. He would do best in a calm, consistent, small environment that is heavily reliant on reinforcement and attention. He needs support that is emotionally neutral toward his challenges but involves humor. Challenging behavioural responses to transitions and unexpected change need to be anticipated and planned for proactively.

Ninth, identification of a syndrome can lead to communication within clinical and medical disciplines and across disciplines to develop greater understanding and more effective treatment strategies. And it may lead to not only clinical and medical collaboration but also to research that can enhance the field and the lives of countless individuals.

Persons with intellectual disabilities are a heterogeneous group. As noted in the above sections, they differ significantly as a group in terms of their socio-environmental needs, and their psychological and biomedical characteristics. Research and practice has however often treated this population as if they were homogeneous. Studies discuss approaches to work with persons with "developmental disabilities", "intellectual disabilities", or "mental retardation", as if the experience of all persons so labeled is the same. Similarly, classrooms and educational ventures are developed for those who are "developmentally disabled" or "mentally retarded", without regard to individual differences. As such, there has been little discrimination made between those who will benefit from certain educational or intervention approaches because of their disability, and those the system has failed to adapt to the person's individualized learning needs.

One aspect of understanding regarding the individualized needs of persons with intellectual disabilities is to understand their diversity by virtue of their genetic makeup. This however should in no way imply that within syndromes people do not differ as well. Individuals with different syndromes are also the composite of different experiences, opportunities, and idiosyncratic features. So, syndromic identification should not replace individualized planning and support, but rather be one piece that aids in our understanding the individual better. Moreover, Adrienne Asch has cautioned that when describing persons with disabilities there is a tendency to focus on the negative biomedically-determined elements; this contrasts to the biopsychosocial approach and is at odds with the disability rights movement that promotes an image of positive attribution (Asch, 1994).

Because there are many similarities within different syndromes, opportunity is provided to share understanding and information regarding how best to provide educational and intervention approaches that maximize skill development. For example people with Williams syndrome typically have very good auditory processing, so books on tape are great for them. This is a great learning approach for this group of individuals. However, in contrast, persons with Fragile X syndrome have very poor and delayed auditory processing that is inconsistent with their overall functioning. Therefore reliance on this approach to learning would be most ineffective. Clinicians working with individuals can share strategies and as a result enhance their ability to effectively support individuals with different needs.

Conferences, research and collaborative efforts can lead to increased understanding and application to the various individuals who experience a similar syndrome.

Table 11 provides some information about common challenges associated with a particular syndrome called Angelman. Research has been able to determine the rate at which certain behaviors occur in this population (i.e., Hyperactivity- 64-100%, Grabbing others- 100%, Frequent smiling- 96-100%, Hand flapping- 84% (excited/ when walking), Inappropriate laughter- 77-91%, Mouthing objects- 75-100%, Sleep disorder- 57-100%). Moreover, effective strategies such as alternative communication boards can be recommended and common medical vulnerabilities can be identified.

Table 11:

Angelman Syndrome

Formerly known as *Happy Puppet Syndrome*

Incidence: 1 in 25,000 live births

Etiology: Deletion of part of maternal copy of chromosome 15q; paternal uniparental disomy; gene mutation

How to test: Methylation Analysis followed by Cytogenetic and molecular testing, if positive

Physical Characteristics	Behavioral Characteristics	Common Medical Vulnerabilities	Cognitive Implications
Jerky, unsteady gait	Happy disposition	Seizures- 90%	*Strengths*
Hypopigmentation	Lack of speech	Seizures become less severe with age and are the only common medical problem; appear between 1 and 3 years of age	Receptive language higher than expressive language
Characteristic facial appearance:	Short attention span		*Weaknesses*
Long face/prominent jaw	Frequent laughter- unprovoked smiling and laughter (unknown if mood-based)		Severe mental delay
Wide mouth		Sleep disorders	Developmental verbal dyspraxia
Protruding tongue	Hyperactivity- 64-100%	Scoliosis	No verbal imitation/sounds/ actions
Microcephaly- small head, with flat back	Grabbing others- 100%	*Strategies*	*Strategies*
Deep-set eyes	Frequent smiling- 96-100%	Encourage physical activity.	Provide alternate communication strategies (i.e., picture exchange/ picture boards)
Tremors (shakiness)- often get diagnosed with ataxic cerebral palsy	Hand flapping- 84% (excited/ when walking)	To avoid contractures, keep active and mobile for as long as possible.	
	Inappropriate laughter- 77-91%	Wheelchair will aid in mobility	
	Mouthing objects- 75-100%		
	Sleep disorder- 57-100%		
	Affinity for wate, shiny objects, and musical toys		

Tenth, individuals with disabilities or carriers of disabling conditions can gain the knowledge to make informed decisions about reproductive counseling.

This last area is one of great controversy. Society is divided on the topic of reproductive counseling, amniocentesis, prevention of birth diversities, and abortion. It is beyond the scope of this chapter to delve into the complexity of these ethical issues. Moreover, such decisions are to a large extent very personal and within the domain of the individual families.

The identification of various syndromes has been scientifically possible for some time. For example, amniocentesis has allowed for early detection of Down Syndrome prior to birth. However in recent years, the Human Genome project has allowed scientists to identify the nature of the genetic code and the location of various diversities. As a result of this project, the exact location of various diversities has been able to be identified the transmission of the syndrome within a families (i.e., Fragile X syndrome). This is the New Genetics (Richards, 1995).

This New Genetics has caused concern for many professionals, advocates, family members and individuals with developmental disabilities (i.e., Rioux, 1996; Ticoll, 1996). The nature of the research may be without bias, however the application of that research can lead to an improvement in the quality of life of individuals affected by the science or a reduction in quality of life or even the elimination of life itself. The field of intellectual disabilities is reasonably worried that this new research be used for the benefit of individuals with disabilities and not become a new Eugenics Movement.

The Eugenics Movement developed into full strength in the early part of the 20th century. It was a movement that was based on the belief that society would be improved if there could be control of genetic planning both for features that were respected (intelligence, height, beauty, health) and for features that were not valued (disability, mental illness, immorality and criminality). This movement quickly moved to selective breeding and population control, which for hundreds of thousands of people with disabilities world-wide eventually led to sterilization and for some, especially in the Nazi regime of Germany, lead to genocide (Scheerenberger, 1983).

As a result of such heinous actions, advocates for persons with disabilities are logically wary of the potential ramifications from the research of the New Genetics Movement. "Reaction against the genetics movement has contributed to the failure to advance further enquiry into behavioural genetics. Moreover, this reluctance is most apparent with respect to the proposition that people with certain genetically determined disabilities might also have been more socially undesirable natural characteristics" (O'Brien & Yule, 1995, p. 8). Advocates have suggested that the "channelling of more and more resources to eliminate disability increases the likelihood of discrimination against people with disabilities" (Rioux, 1996, p. 10). However, a categorical stance on this topic fails to address that an understanding of genetic and chromosomal syndromes can greatly enhance the life of individuals with developmental disabilities. Indeed it can be also misapplied to make eugenic decisions about life itself. Thus the role of careful ethical monitoring of practice becomes paramount.

An example where genetic testing is appropriate is if a mother knows that she is a carrier of PKU. As discussed above, children with PKU do not metabolize the amino acid phenylalanine. By following a specific, phenylalanine-free diet from infancy, the severe/profound intellectual disabilities can be circumvented so that only subtle cognitive and attention problems exist (Waisbren, Brown, de Sonneville, & Levy, 1994). It is important for mothers with PKU to control their diets before conception through to delivery (Cheetham, Gitta, & Morrison, 1999).

Advocates have cautioned that the funding and acceptance of the New Genetics should be based on a fundamental principle that it will NOT be promoted and applied in a way that creates passive Eugenics. "In other words, disability should not be the sole reason for eliminating foetuses any more than we would accept sex or race as a reason for abortion." (Rioux, 1996, p. 7).

The authors of this chapter see the amazing potential of syndromic identification to aid in the quality of life of the individuals with intellectual disabilities, and it is with that purpose that this chapter is dedicated.

Summary

Professionals in the field of developmental disabilities must be in a constant state of learning. In the past decade the field has been expanding exponentially regarding the knowledge of biomedical influences and genetics on behavior. It is now recognized that an individual's development is linked to the integration of a number of biomedical, psychological and social influences (Griffiths et al., 1998). Knowledge gained from understanding syndromes needs to be integrated into our information bank on persons with developmental disabilities if clinicians are truly trying to take a whole person approach to support and intervention.

Glossary of Terms

Adrenarche- *Puberty induced by hyperactivity of the adrenal cortex*

Athetosis- *Condition in which movements are involuntary, slow, squirming, and continuous. These movements occur during flexing, extending, supination (turning the palm up), and pronation (turning the palm down) of the hands and fingers. There may also be a difficulty moving the toes, feet, face, or neck*

Bruxism- *Grinding, gnashing or clenching of the teeth*

Behavioral phenotype- *a characteristic cluster of behaviors that are associated with a specific syndrome. Some of these phenotypes are unusual and unique to the syndrome.*

Coprolalia- *Involuntary use of obscene language or writing*

Copropraxia- *Involuntary bodily response that is either vulgar, sexual, or obscene*

Cryptorchidism- *Failure of testicular descent into the scrotum*

Dyspraxia- *An impairment or immaturity of the organization of movement. Associated with this may be problems of language, perception, and thought*

Echolalia- *Repetition of verbal utterances made by others*

Echopraxia- *Pathological repetition of the actions of other people as if echoing them*

Edema- *Swelling of the soft tissues caused by excess fluid*

Hyperacusis- *Impaired tolerance to normal environmental sounds. Ears lose most of their dynamic range, which is the ability of the ear to deal with quick shifts in sound loudness*

Hypercalcemia- *Excessive blood levels of calcium*

Hyperreflexia- *Reaction of the autonomic (involuntary) nervous system to over-stimulation, which may include high blood pressure, change in heart rate, skin color changes (pallor, redness, blue-grey coloration), and profuse sweating*

Hypertension- *Persistently high arterial blood pressure*

Hypogonadism- *Small testes*

Hypopigmentation- *Decrease in pigment production in hair and skin*

Hypospadias- *Condition where the opening of the penis is found somewhere back along the shaft, anywhere from tip to base, and it is often accompanied by other differences such as penile twisting, a "hooked" appearance because the glans bends down, and a hooded, incomplete foreskin*

Hypotonia- *Decreased muscle tone*

Kyphosis- *Curvature of the spine*

Macrocephaly- *Circumference of the head is larger than established norms for the age and gender of the infant or child*

Macroorchidism- *Enlarged testicles*

Microcephaly- *Circumference of the head is smaller than established norms for the age and gender of the infant or child*

Mitral valve prolapse- *Fairly common and often benign disorder in which a slight deformity of the mitral valve (situated in the left side of the heart) can produce a degree of leakage (mitral insufficiency). Mitral valve prolapse causes a characteristic heart sound (click) that may be heard through a stethoscope.*

Onychotillomania- *Compulsive habit of picking on the cuticles or at the nails*

Otitis media- *Inflammation of the area behind the eardrum*

Peripheral neuropathy- *Medical phrase denoting functional disturbances and/or pathological changes in the peripheral nervous system*

Pica- *Ingestion of non-food items*

Polyembolokoilamania- *Insertion of foreign objects into bodily orifices*

Postaxial polydactyly- *An extra digit is located next to the fifth digit*

Scoliosis- *Curvature of the spine*

Sensory integration- *Disruption in the way the brain processes the intake, organization, and output of information, which can result in hypersensitivity or hyposensitivity to stimuli.*

Strabismus- *Commonly known as crossed-eyes, is a vision condition in which a person cannot align both eyes simultaneously under normal conditions. One or both of the eyes may turn in, out, up or down*

Tactile defensiveness- *Overly sensitive to touch*

Supravalvular aortic stenosis- *Localized narrowing of the aorta above the aortic sinuses*

Resources

Dykens, E.M., Hodapp, R.M., & Finucane, B.M. (2000). *Genetics and intellectual disability syndromes: A new look at behavior and interventions.* Baltimore, MD: Paul H. Brookes.

O'Brien, G. & Yule, W. (1995). *Behavioral phenotypes.* Cambridge: Cambridge University Press.

References

Asch, A. (1994). The human Genome and disability rights. *The Disability Rag and ReSource. January/February*, 345-358.

Cheetham, T., Gitta, M., & Morrison, B. (1999). Some common syndromes associated with developmental disabilities. In I. Brown & M. Percy (Eds.), *Developmental disabilities in Ontario* (pp. 253-272). Toronto, ON: Front Porch Publishing

Dykens, E. M. & Hodapp, R. M. (1997). Treatment issues in genetic mental retardation syndromes. *Professional Psychology: Research and Practice, 28*, 263-270.

Dykens, E. M., Hodapp, R. M., & Finucane, B. M. (2000). *Genetics and intellectual disability syndromes: A new look at behavior and interventions.* Baltimore, MD: Paul H. Brookes.

Flint, J. & Yule, W. (1994). Behavioral phenotypes. In M. Rutter, E. Taylor, & L. Hersov (Eds.), *Child and adolescent psychiatry, 3rd Edition* (pp. 666-687). Oxford: Blackwell Scientific.

Griffiths, D. M., Gardner, W. I., & Nugent, J. (1998). *Behavioral supports: Individual centered interventions. A multimodal functional approach.* Kingston, NY: NADD Press.

Griffiths, D. & Gardner, W. I. (2002). The integrated biosychosocial approach to challenging behaviors. In D. M. Griffiths, C. Stavrakaki, & J. Summers (Eds.), *Dual Diagnosis: An introduction to the mental health needs of persons with developmental disabilities.* Sudbury, ON: Habilitative Mental Health Resource Network.

Hodapp, R. M. (1997). Direct and indirect behavioral effects of different genetic disorders of mental retardation. *American Journal on Mental Retardation*, 102(1), 67-79.

Luria, A. R. (1966). *Human brain and psychological processes*. New York, NY: Harper & Row.

Matalainen, R., Airaksinen, E., Mononen, T., Launiala, K., & Kaarianinen, R. (1995. A population based study on the causes of severe and profound mental retardation. Acta Pediatricia, 84,261-266.

O'Brien, G. & Yule, W. (1995). *Behavioral phenotypes*. Cambridge: Cambridge University Press

Opitz, J.M. (1996). *Historiography of the causal analysis of mental retardation*. Speech to the 29th annual Gatlinburg Conference on Research and Theory in Mental Retardation and Developmental Disabilities. Gatlinburg, TN, March.

Papolos, D.F., Faedda, G.L., Veit, S., Goldbert, R., Morrow, B., Kucherlapati, R., & Shpritzen, R.J. (1998). Bipolar spectrum disorders in patients diagnoses with velo-cardio-facial syndromes: Does a hemizygous deletion on chromosome 22q11 result in bipolar affective disorder? *American Journal of Psychiatry*, *153*, 1541-1547.

Pulver, A.E., Nestadt, G., Shpritzen, R.J., Lamacz, M., Wolyniec, P.S., Morrow, B., Karayiorgou, M., Antonarakis, W.E., Housman, D., & Kucherlapati, R. (1994). Psychotic illness in patients diagnoses with velo-cardio-facial syndrome and their relatives. *Journal of Nervous and Mental Disease*, *182*, 476-478.

Richards, S. (1995). The new genetics. In G. O'Brien & W., Yule (Eds.), *Behavioral Phenotypes* (pp. 24-35) . Cambridge: Cambridge University Press

Rioux, M. (1996). Reproductive technology: A rights issue. *Entourage,* Summer, 5-7

Sacks, O. (1995). *An anthropologist on Mars*. New York: Vintage Books.

Scheerenberger, R.C. (1983). *A history of mental retardation*. Baltimore, MD: Paul H. Brookes.

Ticoll, M. (1996). The human genome project- A challenge for the new millenium. *Entourage,* Summer, 10-12.

Vygotsky, L. (1993). Defect and compensation. In R.W. Rieber & A.S. Croton (Eds.), The collected works of L.S. Vygotsky: Vol. 2. The fundamentals of defectology (pp. 52-64). New York: Plenum (original work published in 1927).

Waisbren, S.E., Brown, M.J., de Sonneville, L.M.J., & Levy, H.L. (1994). Review of neuropsychological functioning in treated phenylketonuria. *Acta Paediatrica* (Suppl 407), 98-103.

Zigler, E., & Hodapp, R.M. (1986). Understanding mental retardation. New York: Cambridge University Press.

CHAPTER 2

Fragile X Syndrome

Tara J. T. Kennedy, Daune MacGregor, Jay Rosenfield

Introduction

The Fragile X syndrome (FXS; other common abbreviations include fra(X) and FraX) is a common genetic cause of developmental disability/mental retardation. Approximately 1 in 4,000 people in the general population are affected by FXS (Turner, Webb, Wake, & Robinson, 1996), while 1 in 259 females and 1 in 700 males are carriers who can pass on the syndrome to their offspring (Rousseau, Morel, Rouillard, Khandjian, & Morgan, 1996). FXS affects cognitive abilities, social interactions, behavior, and physical health. FXS can cause a wide spectrum of symptoms, ranging from mild learning or emotional problems, to moderate or severe developmental disability/mental retardation. Males with the full syndrome are usually the most severely affected, and carriers have mild effects or no effects at all.

The wide variety of symptoms and the effects on each of the biomedical, psychological and social spheres present challenging issues for families, caregivers and individuals whose lives are affected by FXS. This chapter will discuss the genetic cause of FXS, the full spectrum of effects of the syndrome, the principles of a multidisciplinary approach to providing care for people affected by FXS, and sources for further information and support.

Biomedical Features

Genetics

The first description of FXS was in 1943, when Martin and Bell described a family with 11 developmentally disabled males and some mildly affected females (Martin & Bell, 1943). Forty years later, this family was found to have FXS on genetic testing. In the late 1960's, (Lubs, 1969) reported a break, or fragile site, on the lower end of the X chromosome in members of a similar family.This fragile site is called FRAXA, and it is the location of the genetic abnormality associated with FXS. It is now recognized that there are over 100 abnormalities on the X chromosome (called X-linked diseases) which produce developmental disability/mental retardation (Lubs, Schwartz, Stevenson, & Arena, 1996). Two other identified fragile sites on the X chromosome, called FRAXE and FRAXF, are usually associated with milder cognitive impairments (Hagerman, 1999).

Every cell in the body contains chromosomes. Chromosomes are units of genetic material that contain the information needed for our bodies to develop and function. Normally, humans have 23 pairs of chromosomes, or 46 chromosomes in total. The first 22 pairs are the same in males and females. The 23rd pair, the sex chromosomes, is different for males and females. Females have two X chromosomes, while males have an X chromosome and a Y chromosome.

When genetic material is passed on to offspring, only one of each pair of chromosomes is passed on in the egg or the sperm. Thus a female will pass on an X chromosome to all of her offspring, as both of her sex chromosomes are X chromosomes, but a male could pass on either an X or a Y. This concept has major implications for the inheritance pattern and clinical features of FXS. Females with the FXS mutation have one abnormal X chromosome, and one normal X chromosome. The unaffected X chromosome partially compensates for the abnormal one. Thus females usually have milder symptoms than males, who have only the one abnormal X chromosome, and no second normal X chromosome to compensate. Affected females can pass either the normal or the abnormal X chromosome to their offspring, and thus each child has a 50% chance of inheriting the syndrome. Males with FXS will pass their (normal) Y chromosome to each of their sons, who will thus never be affected, and will pass the affected X chromosome to each of their daughters, who will be more mildly affected, but who are at risk for producing offspring with severe FXS. **(Figure 1)**

In 1991, the specific gene on the X chromosome which is responsible for FXS was identified and named FMR1 (Fragile X Mental Retardation-1) (Verkerk et al., 1991). This gene is responsible for producing a protein called FMRP (Fragile X mental retardation protein). The specific function of this protein is not yet well understood, but it may be involved in the process of transmitting messages between different parts of the cell (Kaufmann & Reiss, 1999). It is the absence of FMRP that results in the clinical features of FXS. Individuals who have a less severe abnormality of FMR1 will still produce FMRP, but at lower levels than normal, and will have the milder forms of FXS (Kaufmann, Abrams, Chen, & Reiss, 1999).

Figure 1: Schematic representation of patterns of inheritance of X chromosomes with Fragile X mutation or premutation.

γ = Y chromosome, χ = X chromosome, χ_χ = X chromosome with Fragile X mutation

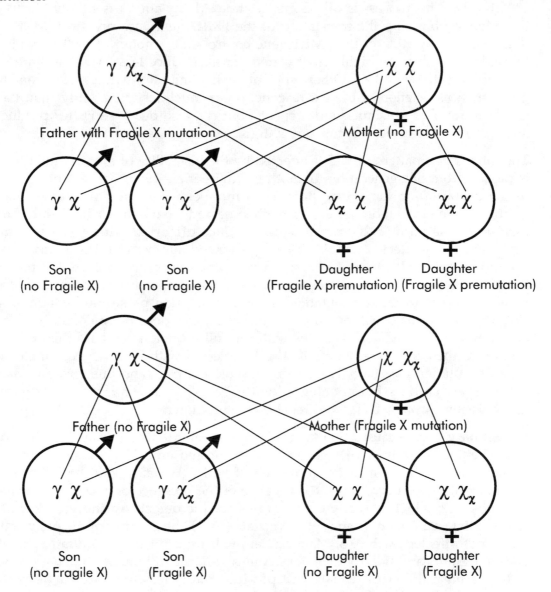

The type of mutation in the FMR1 gene that causes FXS was the first mutation of its type to be discovered (Yu et al., 1991). The initial portion of the FMR1 gene has a sequence of 3 nucleotides (nucleotides are the subunits of genes) that is repeated many times, and is thus called a trinucleotide repeat. The number of repeats in this region varies from 6 to 54 in the normal population (Fu et al., 1991). Individuals who are carriers, but who are not affected by FXS, have between 55 and 200 repeats. This is called a premutation. Individuals with more than 230 trinucleotide repeats have the full mutation, and thus have decreased or absent FMRP production and show the clinical features of FXS.

An abnormally long sequence of trinucleotide repeats (more then 230) in the FMR-1 gene decreases FMRP production by causing extra molecules to be attached to the FMR1 gene. This process is called methylation. Methylation essentially "turns off" the gene, by blocking the translation of the FMR1 gene into protein (FMRP). The degree of methylation of the FMR1 gene controls the amount of FMRP produced: individuals with more highly methylated genes produce less FMRP and are more severely affected with FXS. Other types of genetic mutation which affect the FMR1 gene, such as deletion of the entire gene, occur much less frequently than the increase in number of trinucleotide repeats, but can also decrease FMRP production and produce the clinical features of FXS (Kaufmann & Reiss, 1999).

The inheritance pattern of FXS is affected by the instability of the premutation as it is passed from one generation to another (Nolin et al., 1996). Trinucleotide repeats in the premutation range can increase in number when they are passed from a mother to a child, but do not increase when passed from a father to a child. Thus a carrier female with 55-200 repeats can produce offspring with greater than 230 repeats who are affected with FXS. The greater the number of trinucleotide repeats present on the FMR1 gene of a carrier female, the greater the chance that the number of trinucleotide repeats will expand to a full mutation in her children. Conversely, when a male with the full mutation or the premutation passes on his abnormal X chromosome to his daughters, the number of repeats does not increase in number, and may even be reduced. Females with the full mutation can pass this full mutation on to their offspring, who will also be affected with FXS, whereas males with the full mutation pass on only a premutation size repeat, and thus produce daughters who are carriers, but not affected with FXS. The reasons for the differences in transmission through males and females are unknown.

In summary, FXS is caused by the presence of greater than 230 trinucleotide repeats at the beginning of the FMR1 gene on the X chromosome. This causes methylation of the gene and thus prevents production of FMRP. Females with the full mutation are generally less severely affected because of the presence of a second (normal) X chromosome, which partially compensates for the defect. An individual with an intermediate number of trinucleotide repeats (55-200) is a carrier of the premutation, but is not affected with FXS. Male carriers will transmit the premutation to all of their daughters and none of their sons. Males with the full mutation usually pass on a decreased number of repeats and produce daughters who are carriers of the premutation. Transmission through female carriers of the premutation carries high risk of expansion of the number of trinucleotide repeats, thus producing offspring with the full mutation and clinical signs of FXS. Females with the full mutation have a 50% risk of transmitting FXS to each offspring of either sex.

Case Study

Robert is a 3-year-old boy who was assessed by a general paediatrician because of language difficulties. He was born at full term, with a birthweight of 8 pounds, following a normal pregnancy and delivery. He was a healthy infant, who had excellent growth despite his tendency to spit up after feeding. He had a right-sided inguinal hernia, which was repaired at 12 months of age. He had a "lazy eye", which was treated with patching from 6 months to 18 months with good results. He had frequent ear infections for the first 3 years of life, but his hearing was normal. No other medical problems were identified.

Developmentally, his parents did not have any concerns until the second year of life. Robert learned to walk at 14 months of age, was able to feed himself with a spoon at 18 months of age, and was toilet trained by 30 months. He didn't say his first words, however, until just after his 2nd birthday, and still wasn't combining any words together at 3 years of age. His parents had also noticed that he was lagging behind the other children in motor skills when he started nursery school 3 months prior to his assessment.

On physical examination, Robert's height, weight and head circumference were greater than the 90th percentile ("off the chart") for his age. He was noted to have large, rather prominent ears, but his facial features were not unusual. His general physical examination was normal apart from generally low muscle tone. A developmental screening test revealed that at 36 months of age, Robert's gross motor development was at an 18 month level, while his fine motor and adaptive skills were at a 21 month level. His receptive and expressive language skills were areas of particular difficulty and had reached only the 15 month level.

Because of Robert's developmental problems, a number of tests were ordered, including blood tests for genetic and metabolic problems.

Clinical Features

The physical features of FXS can vary widely depending on the type of defect in the FMR1 gene that is present in an individual, as well as the unique combination of other genetic traits present within any given family. As well, some features can become more prominent with age and thus be absent in young children (Simko, Hornstein, Soukup, & Bagamery, 1989). However, there are a number of physical traits which are typical of individuals with FXS, and which may also be seen, although to a milder degree, in carriers of the premutation (Riddle et al., 1998).

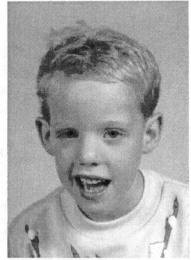

Figure 2
(picture of FXS face)

The classic facial features of FXS include a long face, prominent chin and large, prominent ears with cupping of the upper border. Other facial characteristics present in FXS include a large head with prominent forehead, small eyes, puffiness around the eyes, epicanthic folds (a vertical fold of skin on the inner border of the eye), high arched palate and dental crowding (Hagerman, 1999). **(Figure 2, Table 1)**

Table 1: Typical Facial Features of Fragile X Syndrome

- long face
- prominent chin
- large, prominent ears
- cupped upper border of the ears
- prominent forehead
- small eyes
- epicanthic folds
- high arched palate
- dental crowding

Associated with the changes in facial structure are some specific medical problems. Children with FXS have a particularly high rate of middle ear infections, which can interfere with hearing. Thus speech and language development can be adversely affected if the ear infections are not treated aggressively (Hagerman, Altshul-Stark, & McBogg, 1987). Sinus infections are also relatively common in children with FXS. Problems with snoring are common, and sleep apnea (pauses in breathing during sleep) is seen in a small minority of children (Hagerman, 1999). Abnormalities of the eyes, including abnormal alignment (lazy eye or strabismus) and refractive errors (near or far sightedness), occur in 25% of children with FXS (Hatton, Buckley, Lachiewicz, & Roberts, 1998).

Individuals with FXS have unusually loose and supple supporting tissues (connective tissue dysplasia) which produces skin which is described as soft and velvet-like, and particularly flexible joints. The abnormal connective tissue also leads to higher rates of problems such as flat feet, congenital hip dislocation, other joint dislocations, hernias, and scoliosis (Davids, Hagerman, & Eilert, 1990). The connective tissue of the heart can be affected as well, leading to mitral valve prolapse (a floppy valve between two (2) of the chambers of the heart) and mild dilation of the aorta (the main outflow vessel of the heart). **(Table 2)**

Table 2:   Other Physical Features of Fragile X Syndrome

- large head
- soft skin
- joint flexibility
- low muscle tone
- enlarged testes

Another characteristics feature of males with FXS is enlargement of the testes (testicular volume greater than 30 ml). This process usually begins between 8 and 9 years of age, and is present in 80% of adolescent and adult males with FXS (Butler,

Allen, Haynes, Singh, Watson, & Breg, 1991). Both males and females with FXS are fertile and can produce offspring; however, the likelihood of reproduction is reduced in severely affected individuals with FXS due to the social limitations produced by their cognitive impairment. Some research studies have suggested that female carriers have an increased risk of early menopause and increased frequency of twin pregnancies (Vianna-Morgante, 1999). Timing of puberty is normal in children with FXS, but the pubertal growth spurt is reduced (Loesch, Huggins, & Hoang, 1995). Although children with FXS have a tendency to increased growth, with increased height and weight compared to their peers, the decreased pubertal growth spurt often results in short stature in adulthood.

Neurological abnormalities seen in FXS include low muscle tone (hypotonia) and poor motor coordination, as well as hypersensitivity to visual, auditory, and tactile stimuli. Sleep problems, including decreased total sleep time and increased night wakenings have been documented in children with FXS (Hagerman, 1999). Seizures are seen in 18% of children with FXS, and can be of a variety of types (Musumeci et al., 1999). The seizures associated with FXS are often easily controlled with medication, and are often outgrown by adulthood. Magnetic Resonance Imaging (MRI) scans of the brains of individuals with FXS show a decrease in the size of a part of the brain called the vermis of the cerebellum (Mostofsky, Mazzocco, Aakalu, Warsofsky, Denckla, & Reiss, 1998). The cerebellum is involved with sensory processing, attention and learning, and thus this difference in the structure of the brain may be related to the behavior and cognitive problems seen in FXS (see following sections). **(Table 3, Figure 3)**

Table 3:   Medical Problems Associated with Fragile X Syndrome

Head and neck:
   ♦ middle ear infections
   ♦ sinus infections
   ♦ snoring and sleep apnea
   ♦ abnormal eye alignment
   ♦ near or far sightedness

Musculoskeletal:
   ♦ joint dislocations
   ♦ flat feet
   ♦ scoliosis

Cardiovascular:
   ♦ mitral valve prolapse
   ♦ dilation of the aorta

Nervous system:
   ♦ seizures

Case Study

Discussion of Robert's family history revealed that big ears were considered a family trait on his mother's side. Robert had a 6-year-old sister, Jane, who had generalized seizures since 2 years of age, and was on an anti-seizure medication. She had not been noted to have had delayed development as a young child, but was having significant difficulty in Grade 1. She was not yet able to print her name or to count past 10. Robert's parents were both healthy and had completed high school with no particular learning problems. His mother had just discovered that she was pregnant for the third time. The only other family history of note was that Robert had a female cousin, Anne, the daughter of his mother's sister, who was in a special education class at school and was noted at family gatherings to be hyperactive.

The results of Robert's blood tests revealed that he was affected with Fragile X Syndrome (FXS). He was found to have 700 trinucleotide repeats at the beginning of the FMR1 gene. His family was given information regarding the diagnosis and was told of the Fragile X Foundation chapter in their local area. Robert was referred for speech and language therapy, physiotherapy and occupational therapy. He was also referred for a cardiac assessment, which was normal.

Robert's family was referred to a genetics clinic, where they met with a genetic counselor and a medical geneticist. After further discussion, other family members were tested for FXS. Robert's mother was found to be a carrier of the premutation, with 120 trinucleotide repeats on one X chromosome, and 30 repeats on the other. His older sister, Jane, was also found to be affected with FXS, having 610 trinucleotide repeats at the beginning of the FMR1 gene on one X chromosome, and 12 repeats on the other. Robert's mother had an amniocentesis and found that the unborn baby, a girl, was not affected with FXS. Later, extended family members were also tested for FXS. Robert's maternal grandfather and aunt and one female cousin were found to be carriers of the premutation. His cousin Anne was found to have FXS. Figure 3(pedigree)

Diagnosis

FXS is diagnosed by genetic testing performed on a blood sample taken at any age, or on cells obtained early in pregnancy by amniocentesis or chorionic villus sampling. The test is specific for the abnormality of the FMR1 gene, and can detect the number of trinucleotide repeats that is present, thus identifying both premutation carriers and individuals with the full mutation. Testing for FXS done prior to the early 1990's, before the FMR1 gene was discovered, could detect abnormalities, called fragile sites, of the X chromosome in the FMR1 region, but was not specific for FXS (Turner et al., 1996).

Testing for FXS should be performed on children and adults with developmental disability/mental retardation of unknown etiology (Brown et al., 1996). Children with milder learning problems and physical and/or behavioral features (see following sections) typical of FXS should also be tested. A number of clinical checklists have been developed to screen for patients who are at particularly high risk (Hagerman, Amiri, & Cronister, 1991). Consideration should also be given to potential alternative or co-existing diagnoses such as Prader-Willi syndrome, Tourette's syndrome (see Chapter 9), or Klinefelter syndrome (males with an extra X chromosome).

Figure 3: Pedigree of Robert (Case Study example). The numbers below the names and symbols represent the number of trinucleotide repeats on the X chromosomes (one for each male and two for each female).

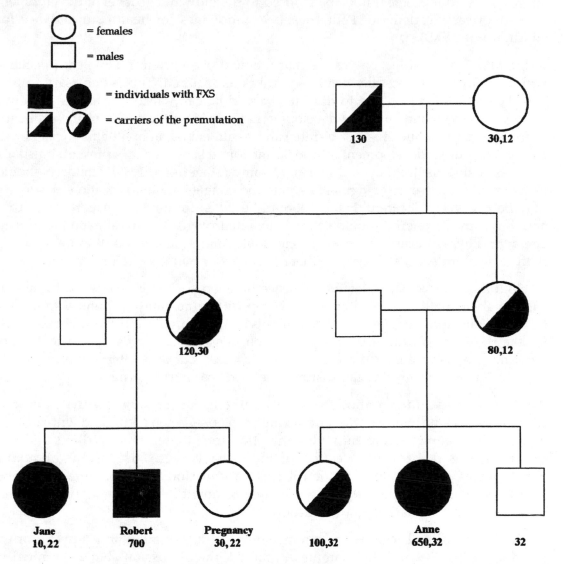

Once a diagnosis of FXS is made, a detailed family history is necessary in order to identify other family members who may be affected by FXS or who may be premutation carriers, in order to offer them testing for this condition. A genetic counselor should be involved in this process, to educate families about the transmission patterns of FXS and the wide spectrum of clinical involvement. The counselor is also a source of support and information during the process of notifying other family members who may be affected, as this can be difficult and frightening for families. An ongoing relationship with a genetic counselor is important for families affected by FXS, as they provide links to support groups and information about options for family members contemplating pregnancy (Staley-Gane, Flynn, Neitzel, Cronister, & Hagerman, 1996).

Management of Medical Issues

A number of the medical issues arising in FXS require specific management and surveillance. Management must be tailored to the individual's level of development (see American Academy of Pediatrics 1996 guidelines for health surveillance for children with FXS).

In the first 2 years of life, aggressive management of recurrent middle ear infections with antibiotics, and possibly ventilation tubes, is required. This is necessary to prevent hearing difficulties due to fluid in the middle ear, which can have a negative impact on speech and language development. Early identification of visual problems or misalignment of the eyes (strabismus) and treatment by an ophthalmologist is necessary for optimal development of visual function. If sleep apnea is present, it usually resolves with tonsillectomy and adenoidectomy (Hagerman, 1999). Children should be assessed for presence of inguinal hernias and congenital hip dislocation, as surgery may be necessary. A careful history should be taken for any suggestion of seizures and, if positive, a referral should be made to a neurologist for investigation and management. Physical examination of the cardiovascular system should occur regularly with referral for echocardiogram if there are signs of mitral valve prolapse.

In childhood, surveillance for the presence of sleep problems, seizure activity and cardiac abnormalities should continue. Sleep difficulties may respond to administration of melatonin (Hagerman, 1999). In this age group, children should be assessed for the presence of orthopedic problems such as scoliosis and flat feet. These problems may, on occasion, require orthopedic assessment and intervention, such as orthotics, when significant gait disturbance or discomfort is produced.

Adolescents and adults continue to require surveillance for seizure activity and cardiac problems. Individuals with mitral valve prolapse, when associated with leakage of the valve, require treatment with antibiotics prior to dental procedures and certain surgeries to prevent infection of the heart valves. Discussions of sexual development, fertility and birth control, and transmission of FXS are important, and should occur in a supportive and relaxed environment in language appropriate for the affected individual's cognitive level.

Medical professionals can be an ongoing source of information and support for individuals with FXS and their families. Although the discussion above is limited to medical issues, physicians and other medical professionals must be involved in the management of the psychological and social aspects of FXS as described in the following sections.

Common Myths

1 *Females cannot have FXS*

Because FXS is an X-linked disorder, many people believe that it can not affect females, assuming that the normal X chromosome would completely compensate for the chromosome carrying the mutation. While all females do have two X chromosomes, only one of them is active in each cell in the body. So one of the two X chromosomes is inactivated in every cell. The percentage of cells in which the normal X chromosome is the active one is called the activation ratio. The higher the activation ratio, the more FMRP will be produced, and the milder the FXS symptoms will be. Symptoms of FXS in females depend on how many cells have an active normal X chromosome, especially in important parts of the body like the brain. Because of the inactivation of the normal X chromosome in some of the cells of the body, the normal X chromosome cannot compensate fully for the affected X chromosome, and females with the full mutation can indeed have FXS. The presence of the normal X chromosome does, however, account for the fact that females with FXS, as a group, are less severely affected than are males, as some of their cells do produce FMRP. The variation in the activation ratio accounts for the wide variation of symptoms, from mild to severe, in affected females (Riddle et al., 1998).

2 *Individuals who don't exhibit the classic physical features of FXS (protuberant ears, long face, large testes) cannot be affected with the syndrome*

Although the classic features of FXS are widely recognized, many affected individuals are not noted to have many of the classic features, particularly in childhood. Most of the facial features are not apparent until after puberty in many people with FXS. The same is true for the increase in testicular volume, which doesn't begin until age 8 or 9 years, and is most obvious after puberty. Another reason for lack of identification of the facial features is that traits like a long face or large chin are relatively common in the general population, and are present in many people without FXS. Thus subtle facial characteristics of FXS might not be recognized as being caused by this condition until after the diagnosis is made, as many people with FXS do not look particularly unusual. A third reason for the lack of classic features in some individuals with FXS is related to the wide spectrum of severity seen in FXS, due to variation in genetic factors described above such as the activation ratio in females, the degree of methylation of the FMR1 gene, and level of production of FMRP (Hagerman, 1999).

Psychological Features

Case Study

Shortly after school entry, at age 6 years, Robert had a full neuropsychological assessment. Overall, Robert's cognitive abilities were found to be below the first (lowest) percentile for his age on the Stanford-Binet Intelligence Scale- Fourth Edition (Thorndike, Hagen, & Sattler,1986). This placed him in the range of moderate developmental disability. Robert had relative strengths in the skills tested by the pattern analysis subtest (replicating two-dimensional patterns) and the absurdities subtest (visually detecting and describing problems in pictures). He had particular difficulty in the memories for sentences subtest, which is a test of auditory memory. On the Wide Range Assessment of Memory and Learning, Robert showed much better performance on the Story Memory subtest (recalling details from a story) than on the Verbal Learning subtest (recalling lists of words). This indicated that Robert was better able to retain information presented in a meaningful format, such as a story. On the Vineland Adaptive Behavior Scale (Sparrow, Balla, & Cicchetti,1984) (a semi-structured parental interview), Robert showed relative strengths in the domains of daily living skills and socialization.

Early Development

Early developmental milestones are delayed in children with FXS. A study of males with the full mutation showed that, in the first three years of life, development progressed at approximately half the rate that would be expected in children with typical development (Bailey, Hatton, & Skinner, 1998). Delayed onset of language is common in children with FXS, with expressive abilities being more delayed than receptive abilities. Mild delays are seen in gross motor skills, with particular difficulties in skills requiring coordination, such as riding a bicycle. Children with FXS often have relative strengths in fine motor skills and manual dexterity, but have difficulty with tasks requiring integration of visual information with motor output, resulting in poor printing and cutting skills. Children (and adults) with FXS show particular strengths in the areas of personal care and domestic skills (Friefeld, MacGregor, & Silverstein, 1991).

Cognitive Effects

The degree of cognitive involvement in FXS covers a wide spectrum. The level of cognitive impairment is related to the type and degree of abnormality of the FMR1 gene (Tassone et al., 1999). Males with a full mutation and a fully methylated FMR1 gene have cognitive abilities in the moderate to severe range of developmental disability/mental retardation (Merenstein, Sobesky, Taylor, Riddle, Tran, & Hagerman, 1996). Approximately 13% of males with the full mutation are described as "high-functioning": they have cognitive abilities which are above the developmentally disabled range (i.e.: borderline or average cognitive abilities) (Hagerman et al., 1994). The high functioning males with the full mutation have similar areas of cognitive weakness and behavioral difficulty as do other males with FXS, but to a lesser degree.

The level of cognitive impairment in females with the full FXS mutation is related to the percentage of cells in which the normal X chromosome is active (activation ratio) (Riddle et al., 1998), as well as to the level of methylation of the FMR1 gene and amount of FRMP production. Of females with a full mutation, 50-70% have cognitive abilities in the developmental disability range (deVries et al., 1996). The remainder has more subtle learning problems and difficulties with executive function abilities (attention, planning, organization, working memory, inhibition). Carriers of the premutation generally have cognitive abilities in the average range, but can have learning disabilities and some of the behavioral and emotional characteristics described in a following section.

The cognitive profile in FXS involves weaknesses in processing and remembering auditory information, and in processing abstract or complex information (Freund & Reiss, 1991). Another area of difficulty is visual-motor integration. Strengths include processing of visual information (Kemper, Hageman, & Altshul-Stark, 1988) and memory for visually presented, meaningful information. Individuals with FXS are better at processing information simultaneously than at dealing with long sequences of information. They also perform better when tested on information learned from the environment than on tasks requiring novel problem-solving skills. Academic testing reveals particularly low scores on arithmetic subtests (Hodapp, Leckman, Dykens, Sparrow, Zelinsky, & Ort, 1992). In summary, individuals with FXS respond better to visual than to auditory information, can recall concrete, meaningful material better than abstract or non-contextual material, and are better at imitating and performing practical tasks than at solving new problems. **(Tables 5 & 6)**

A decline in cognitive abilities or IQ scores is seen over time in approximately 30% of individuals with FXS (Wright-Talamante, Cheema, Riddle, Luckey, Taylor, & Hagerman, 1996). This does not represent a loss of skills, but rather a plateau of abilities at mid to late childhood, when abstract reasoning skills fail to progress. This decline in cognitive skills is not seen in more mildly affected individuals.

Language and Communication

The speech of individuals with FXS is often cluttered (fast speech with erratic rhythm) and difficult to understand. Articulation difficulties can be seen and are related to oral motor coordination problems. Patterns of language that are common in FXS include perseveration on phrases and topics, difficulty with pragmatics (use of language for communication and conversation), and poor topic maintenance (Abeduto & Hagerman, 1997). Approximately 11% of males with FXS are non-verbal at age 5 years of age, and these boys tend to have more severe cognitive and physical involvement, as well (Hagerman, 1999).

Case Study

In the school setting, Robert had some significant problems with his behavior. He was described as distractible by his teacher, and was often out of his seat and disturbing other children in the class. He was also having frequent temper tantrums, usually related to changes in routine. He would become extremely upset each time the fire alarm would sound, and would then be unable to calm down sufficiently to participate in his work for the rest of the day. He was noted to have poor eye contact, and his teacher reported that he had difficulty joining in with the other children during recess and lunch hour.

After the neuropsychological assessment, the school psychologist, special education teacher, Grade 1 classroom teacher, and the school principal met with Robert's parents to discuss his behavior problems. Multiple strategies were implemented, including the provision of a 1-on-1 educational assistant in the classroom. Robert was provided with a schedule of daily activities, with a picture of each activity. His educational assistant provided him with 10 and 5-minute warnings of all transitions between activities. Robert was permitted a short break to play with a favorite toy at his desk after each 5 minute interval of quiet work, and longer breaks at an activity centre every 30 minutes. At the earliest sign that Robert was becoming upset, his educational assistant would remove him from the classroom to an adjoining room where he would listen to his favorite audiotape, in an attempt to prevent escalation of his behavior. When Robert's behavior was unacceptable (usually physical aggression during a tantrum), he was removed from his seat to a "time out" corner for a specified period of time. On the playground, Robert was linked with a group of volunteer "buddies" from the Grade 5 and 6 classes, one of whom would accompany Robert outside each day and help him to interact with the other children, providing suggestions and guidance in the social setting.

These interventions made a significant difference in Robert's behavior initially. In later grades, Robert's distractibility and impulsivity continued to cause significant problems in the classroom. After further assessment by his pediatrician, he was started on low-dose methylphenidate (Ritalin ™), which did produce an improvement in his ability to focus on his work. Helping Robert to control his behavior remained a significant issue throughout his school years, which required frequent input from family and professionals to produce effective, evolving behavior management strategies.

Behavioral Effects

The behavioral effects of FXS, like the physical and cognitive effects, cover a wide spectrum. Some behavioral traits vary with gender and with degree of genetic abnormality. The behavioral manifestations of FXS can be a significant source of stress for families and caregivers, and are an important area on which to focus intervention and treatment efforts.

A characteristic behavioral trait of males with FXS is distractibility, associated with a short attention span. This is seen in almost all males with a full mutation. In addition, hyperactivity is seen in 80% of boys and 35% of girls with FXS (Hagerman, 1999). Many children with FXS will meet criteria for attention deficit hyperactivity disorder (ADHD) on formal assessment (Baumgardner, Reiss, Freund, & Abrams, 1995). This hyperactivity and distractibility can interfere significantly with learning and cause disruption in both the school and home settings.

Another characteristic of many children with FXS is hypersensitivity to sound, touch, smell, taste, and visual stimulation (Miller et al., 1999). This hypersensitivity can cause children to become irritated by stimuli that would not be expected to bother other children, such as the textures of certain clothing, or the sound of the vacuum cleaner. Hypersensitivity to stimuli can also cause children to become overwhelmed in crowded, noisy or active situations, and this can lead to frequent and severe temper tantrums.

Other behaviors commonly seen in FXS include hand flapping, hand biting and other hand mannerisms, avoidance of eye contact, and a tendency to perseverate in language and in activities. Although these behaviors are also seen in children with autism spectrum disorders, most children with FXS do not have autism. However, approximately 16% of children with FXS have deficiencies in reciprocal social interaction and show restrictive and repetitive behaviors to a level that meet criteria for diagnosis of autism spectrum disorders (Baumgardner et al., 1995). This incidence of autism spectrum disorders is much higher than in the general population, and children with FXS should be followed with this in mind (Feinstein & Reiss, 1998).

One behavioral feature that is more typical of females with FXS is shyness or social anxiety. Although boys with FXS also feel social anxiety, it can be masked by their hyperactivity. Severe anxiety is seen in up to 40% of females with the full mutation (Lachiewicz & Dawson, 1994) and many can be diagnosed with avoidant personality disorder (social discomfort, aversion to social interaction and fear of rejection) (Freund, Reiss, & Abrams, 1993). Other psychiatric disorders which can be associated with FXS include affective disorders such as depression and bipolar disorder (manic-depression), obsessive-compulsive disorder, and, rarely, psychosis (Hagerman, 1999).

Table 4: Behavioral Characteristics of Fragile X Syndrome

- ♦ distractibility
- ♦ hyperactivity
- ♦ hypersensitivity to stimuli
- ♦ social anxiety

Case Study

During one follow-up visit with Robert's pediatrician, his mother became tearful during a discussion of Robert's social struggles at school. She revealed that her daughter Jane, who was having significantly less severe problems with her academic work than was Robert, was however having difficulty "fitting in", and was very shy. Robert's mother said that she knew that Jane had inherited her shyness from her mother, because she herself had difficulty in social situations. She stated that she usually avoided any social events apart from family gatherings because of the anxiety and stress they produced. She asked for help for her daughter, who was frequently crying at home after school.

Jane was enrolled in a social skills group to help develop strategies to use in a variety of social interactions. She also began to attend an after-school activity group and became a member of the Girl Guides (a group for school-age girls emphasizing recreational and community service activities), which provided social interactions in more structured settings. Jane and her mother had some sessions with a counselor regarding this problem, which they both described as helpful.

Management of Behavioral Features

Strategies for management of inattention, distractibility and hyperactivity include behavioral techniques, educational interventions, and medication. Behavioral approaches include positive reinforcement programs for appropriate behavior, and consistent limit setting. These techniques are also effective in management of other behavioral problems such as temper tantrums. Educational modifications such as preferential seating at the front of the classroom, highly structured schedules, minimization of distractions and breaking down tasks into small, manageable portions can significantly improve performance in the school setting (Spiridigliozzi et al., 1997). If, with these techniques in place, distractibility and hyperactivity continue to be disruptive to learning and social interactions, stimulant medications, most commonly methylphenidate (or Ritalin™) can be added to the treatment regimen. These medications have the effect of helping children to focus on the task at hand and decrease impulsiveness. Children with FXS may be particularly sensitive to the effects of these medications, and should be started initially on a low dose (Hagerman, 1999). Children on stimulant medication need to be monitored carefully for side effects, most commonly decreased appetite and sleep disturbance. Some children with FXS are thought to have improved behavior following folic acid supplementation, or a variety of other complementary therapies (such as special diets). However, research studies have not consistently supported the benefits of folic acid or complementary therapies in FXS (Hagerman, 1996).

Management of hyperreactivity to stimulation includes minimization of overwhelming stimuli in the environment, and advance notice and preparation for transitions to a new environment or activity. Calming interventions (such as music, a favorite video or massage) which are effective for a particular child should be identified and utilized at the first sign that a child is becoming upset. Occupational or other therapists may use sensory integration techniques (such as brushing or deep pressure) to help children with FXS cope with sensory input (Spiridigliozzi et al., 1997). Any child with FXS who is seen to have particular difficulties with reciprocal social interactions, along with communication limitations and restrictive interests or repetitive behaviors, should be referred to an experienced professional in the field of autism spectrum disorders for formal assessment.

The social anxiety seen frequently in FXS requires a multimodal approach. Interventions in the school setting such as a buddy system where a child volunteer accompanies the child with FXS into the schoolyard can provide reassurance and modeling of appropriate social interactions. Social skills groups can provide children with suggestions for behavioral strategies to apply in a variety of social situations and allow them to practice these strategies in a comfortable setting. Medication can be useful in treatment of significant anxiety. The one class of medication used for this purpose is the selective serotonin reuptake inhibitors (SSRI's), such as Prozac™ or Luvox™. Although SSRI's are known as antidepressant medications, they are also useful for the treatment of anxiety, mood lability, obsessive-compulsive behaviors and aggression, which can all be seen in FXS (Hagerman, 1999). Recently, caution has been advised for use of these medications in children under the age of 18 years.

Management of the psychological features of FXS must involve an integrated, multidisciplinary approach. Health care professionals from a variety of disciplines, family members, other caregivers and teachers should collaborate to determine goals of treatment and preferred management strategies. Specific educational interventions, which are critical in the management of the cognitive and behavioral effects of FXS, are discussed in the following sections.

Common Myths

1 *All individuals with FXS are severely developmentally disabled/mentally retarded*

Although the typical male with a full mutation and full methylation of the FMR1 gene has a moderate to severe developmental disability/mental retardation, there is a wide spectrum of cognitive involvement (Merenstein et al., 1996). Males with a full mutation but less than 50% methylation of the FMR1 gene have less cognitive involvement, and can have abilities in the average range. Females with a full mutation have partial compensation for the defect by their second X chromosome, and can have intellectual capacities in the borderline or average ranges in up to 50% of cases (deVries et al., 1996).

2 *Carriers of the fragile X premutation have no clinical effects*

Although many carriers of the FXS premutation have no identifiable effects, recent research suggests that some premutation carriers may have certain characteristics which are related to their carrier status. Although FXS carriers do not have severe cognitive involvement, they may have more subtle learning problems or learning disabilities. Premutation carriers occasionally show very subtle facial characteristics of FXS (like prominent ears)(Riddle et al., 1998). They may have a higher risk than other women for premature ovarian failure and twin pregnancies (Vianna-Morgante, 1999). As well, premutation carriers may be affected by emotional and psychiatric problems such as social phobia, anxiety, depression, or mood swings. These problems have been shown to occur in premutation carriers, who are often mothers of children with FXS, at higher rates than can be attributed to the family stress associated with raising a child with special needs (Franke et al., 1998).

Social Features

Case Study

A number of strategies were utilized in the school setting in attempt to maximize Robert's learning. In the primary grades, he was integrated, for half-days, into the regular classroom setting with a full-time educational assistant and significant modification of the academic work. The other half of the day was spent in a special education classroom with a low teacher-to-student ratio, where he received intensive instruction to develop his pre-reading skills. He was also able to use the computer in the special education classroom, which was his favorite activity. He was withdrawn from the classroom setting on a weekly basis for speech and language therapy and occupational therapy. These therapists also consulted to the classroom. Robert responded best to information relating to pictures or concrete objects, and required frequent visual cueing in order to be able to follow instructions. He could remember new information best when it was related to cars, an area of special interest.

Education

The cognitive, behavioral and physical effects of FXS present a number of challenges in the domain of education. As in the medical and psychological management of FXS, a multidisciplinary approach is necessary in order to address the wide spectrum of issues that can impact on the learning of affected individuals. Assessment of each child's cognitive strengths (Table 5) and weaknesses (Table 6) is necessary for optimal academic planning, and is best achieved through a broad range of standardized neuropsychological measures (Friefeld et al., 1993). Periodic reassessment of goals, academic progress and level of special service provision is necessary for each child with FXS, as their needs can change over time.

Table 5: Cognitive strengths in Fragile X Syndrome
- Recognizing visual information
- Simultaneous processing
- Object memory
- Imitation
- Daily living skills

Table 6: Cognitive Weaknesses in Fragile X Syndrome
- Auditory memory
- Sequential processing
- Abstract reasoning
- Visual-motor integration
- Novel problem solving

The process of educational intervention should begin once a diagnosis of FXS is made, as early as infancy. An infant stimulation program, often involving a physiotherapist, occupational therapist and/or early childhood educator, can help address the gross motor delays, hypotonia, and other developmental delays that are frequently seen in FXS. As a child with FXS progresses into the toddler and early childhood years, intervention should expand to include behavioral strategies to address issues such as temper tantrums and toilet learning (Hagerman, 1999).

Speech and language therapy should begin as soon as problems are identified. A program of exercises can be used to address oral motor incoordination or weakness, which affects articulation. Speech and language therapy can also work on building vocabulary and concept formation. The strength in imitative abilities seen in many children with FXS allows modeling of slow, smooth speech to be an effective technique to help with fluency (Scharfenaker, O'Connor, Stackhouse, Braden, Hickman, & Gray, 1996). Improvement in pragmatics (the social and conversational uses of language) can occur through group speech and language therapy, using techniques such as role-playing and reciprocal conversation exercises (Friefeld et al., 1993). For the children with FXS who have severe expressive language deficits, augmentative communication techniques such as picture communication systems and computer-assisted language output systems can provide an effective means through which to interact with the world around them.

Upon entry into the school system, individualized assessment of the needs of each child with FXS is important for intervention planning. A multidisciplinary approach involving professionals such as special education teachers, psychologists, occupational therapists and speech and language therapists should continue through the school years. It is important that all professionals working with a child with FXS understand the particular learning style associated with the syndrome. Extra training and education sessions for school staff may be required to achieve this understanding (York, von Fraunhofer, Turk, & Sedgwick, 1999).

Consideration must be given to the appropriate classroom placement for a child with FXS. Children with FXS do well in a classroom environment that is as free from distraction as possible, and benefit from small group teaching that allows for frequent repetition and individualized programming and attention. However, children with FXS also benefit from social interactions with peers, who can model appropriate social behaviors. Some children with FXS require an educational assistant to work with them in large group situations to improve understanding of tasks, provide modification of assignments and provide support and suggestions for social interactions. A combination of one-on-one or small group settings with integration into a regular classroom for part of the school day is often the best educational placement option for children with FXS (Spiridigliozzi et al., 1997).

A number of strategies can be employed in the classroom in order to provide an optimal setting for learning for children with FXS (Wilson, Stackhouse, O'Connor, Scharfenaker, & Hagerman, 1994). The establishment of a classroom environment which is as free from overstimulating materials and activity as possible will help distractible and inattentive children to focus on their work. Frequent breaks for physical activity are also helpful. Provision of a predictable, structured daily routine, with visual reminders and advanced warnings of upcoming activities can help children with FXS to deal with transitions. Behavior problems in the classroom can be minimized with a set of consistent expectations and much positive reinforcement for appropriate behaviors and interactions. Children with FXS respond best to information presented visually, and therefore visual aides, pictures, and gestures should be used as often as possible to enhance delivery of new information. Presenting information in a familiar context, relating lessons to areas of particular interest to the child, and modeling to make use of the imitation strengths of children with FXS are also effective teaching strategies. Computers can be very useful in the classroom to enhance communication, circumvent fine motor difficulties with handwriting, provide visual and auditory input, reinforce information in any academic area, and enhance self-esteem. Children with FXS can have relative strengths in computer skills (Hagerman, 1999). See Table 7.

Table 7: Educational Interventions for Students with Fragile X Syndrome

♦ Individualized programming

♦ Reduction of distractions

♦ Frequent repetition

♦ Use of modeling

♦ Structured routine

♦ Frequent breaks

♦ Visual cues and prompts

♦ Concrete examples

Case Study

Upon entry into High School, Robert was placed in a special education classroom with a particular emphasis on life-skills training, and he continued to be integrated into the regular classroom for non-academic subjects. His family was also able to hire a child care worker to spend 8 hours a week with Robert, working on practical skills in the community setting. Robert began to make some sexually inappropriate comments at school and at home. He was enrolled in a group at a local developmental centre designed to explore sexual issues with developmentally disabled adolescents. He and his family also attended a number of sessions with a psychologist to address these issues. In his second year of high school, a vocational training program was added to Robert's curriculum at school. His family was able to meet with a caseworker at the local Association for Community Living to discuss future options for community support for Robert, including group home placement.

Vocational Training

Individuals with FXS should be involved with vocational training by early to mid-adolescence. Their relative strength in learning practical, adaptive skills is a benefit in vocational training. General principles similar to classroom interventions are effective in job training programs. Individuals with FXS do best in work environments that are free of overstimulating inputs such as flashing lights, loud noises, crowded conditions, high levels of activity and strong smells. A structured routine and frequent breaks are helpful to the employee with FXS. Specific hands-on training programs in the work setting, with opportunities for trainers to model required tasks are the most effective training methods for individuals with FXS (Wilson et al., 1994).

Socio-environmental Supports

The level of socio-environmental supports required by individuals with FXS depends largely on the level of cognitive impairment. FXS does not cause physical impairments that necessitate the use of assistive devices or produce barriers to access. Individuals with severe expressive language deficits require augmentative communication devices in order to interact best with others. People with moderate or severe developmental disability/mental retardation require socio-environmental supports ranging from assistance in all daily living skills to supervised independent living. Because of the relative strength seen in the area of adaptive skills, individuals with FXS often require a lesser degree of support in daily activities than do individuals with other disorders at the same cognitive level.

Individuals with FXS who have lesser degrees of cognitive impairment also have requirements for support. Counseling and social skills training can be helpful in management of social anxiety. Parents of children with FXS need information about the syndrome, coordinated care from health and education professionals, access to advocacy and support groups and genetic counseling. Because fertility is generally unimpaired in FXS, all affected individuals require education regarding sexuality issues and contraception. An individual who is familiar with the genetic basis of FXS and transmission risks should provide this information. Extra support and information is required when a pregnancy is being considered or an unexpected pregnancy is discovered (McConkie-Rosell, Robinson, Wake, Staley, Heller, &

Cronister, 1995). Some families affected by FXS have joined together to form support and advocacy groups (see resources).

Common Myths

1 *Many children with FXS also have autism*

Children with FXS often display behaviors such as avoidance of eye contact, hand-flapping and a tendency to perseverate (or get "stuck") on topics of conversation or activities. These behaviors are also common in children with autism spectrum disorders. However, children with autism also have deficits in reciprocal communication and social interactions, as well as unusual repetitive behaviors and sensory interests that are not present in most children with FXS. The avoidance of eye contact and hand mannerisms seen in FXS are thought to be associated with social anxiety and hypersensitivity to sensory input. Children and adults with FXS have been noted to exhibit a particular greeting behavior characterized by turning the head and the upper body away from a partner while shaking hands (Wolff, Gardner, Paccia, & Lappen, 1989), which may be another indication of social anxiety. Although most children with FXS don't have autism, the incidence of autism in individuals with FXS (approximately 15%, although the estimates vary, depending on the method used for diagnosing autism) is still higher than in the general population (Feinstein & Reiss, 1998). Children with FXS who exhibit particular difficulty with social interactions or reciprocal communication should be assessed by a professional with experience in the diagnosis of autism spectrum disorders.

2 *Males with FXS can never have children*

Although FXS affects the growth of the testes, the fertility of males with FXS is generally unimpaired. Males with FXS have been known to produce offspring. However, the likelihood of becoming sexually active is decreased for severely affected males with FXS, because of their social and cognitive deficits (Hagerman, 1999). Sensitive delivery of information regarding sexuality, including genetic implications for potential offspring, is an important part of the education process for all adolescent males with FXS. This information must be communicated in a manner that is tailored to the cognitive level of the affected young man.

Current Trends

Exciting research is ongoing in the FXS field. Current projects include attempts to determine the specific functions of the protein which is deficient in FXS (FMRP), and the specific locations in the body where its effects are most crucial. Experimental approaches to increase the production of FRMP are being studied, including attempts to reverse the methylation process that specifically inhibits FRMP production. The major difficulty with this approach is that it is not yet known how to direct the reversal of methylation so that it affects only the FMR-1 gene. Replacement of the deficient protein is another potential treatment under study, but administration of FRMP to children or adults who already have structural and functional brain and tissue abnormalities may not be of benefit. Optimal protein replacement therapy would involve delivery of FMRP to the fetus in order to prevent structural abnormalities in the brain as it develops, but this is currently technically impossible (McCabe, de la Cruz, & Clapp, 1999).

As the gene responsible for FXS has been identified, gene therapy techniques are being considered as a future possibility, as for many other genetic disorders. To date attempts to have genes successfully inserted into the human genetic code and translated into useful proteins have been unsuccessful, but studies in many genetic disorders are ongoing (Hagerman, 1999).

Neither protein nor gene replacement therapy is likely to be a practical reality for a number of years, but current research is also focused on improving the treatments that are available today. Studies to determine which of the many available medications are the most successful in treating symptoms such as inattention, hyperactivity and anxiety in individuals with FXS are important, as are studies of the specific medication side effect profiles in this population. New developments in educational computer programs are providing extra stimulation and new learning opportunities for children with FXS in the classroom. Screening tests for FXS are being developed which may allow testing for FXS in the general population, and thus better identification of affected families and earlier initiation of counseling and treatment (Hagerman, 1999).

The expansion of knowledge in the field of FXS in the decade since the identification of the responsible gene has been exponential. The potential for similar advances in the years to come is an exciting prospect for families and professionals alike.

Summary

The Fragile X syndrome is a genetic disorder that has physical, cognitive, behavioral and social effects. The syndrome is caused by an abnormality of the FMR1 gene on the X chromosome. The syndrome can be transmitted to offspring of either sex from mothers with FXS or mothers who are carriers. Affected fathers pass the carrier status on to their daughters only. Genetic counseling is important for all affected families.

Individuals with FXS display a wide spectrum of involvement, from mild emotional changes to severe developmental disability. Typical physical characteristics of FXS include a long face, protuberant ears and a prominent chin. Common medical complications include recurrent ear infections, eye misalignment and need for glasses, joint dislocations and seizures. Cognitive effects range from mild to severe, with relative strengths in integration of visual information and learning adaptive skills, and particular weaknesses in auditory memory, sequential processing and abstract thinking. Behavioral traits frequently seen in FXS include distractibility, hyperactivity, hyperreactivity to stimulation and social anxiety.

Management of the many and varied issues which are important to individuals with FXS and their families requires an integrated, multidisciplinary approach. Collaboration between individuals with FXS, their families and caregivers, medical and allied health professionals, educators and social support services is crucial in order to identify important issues, develop management plans, and integrate interventions across domains and contexts. Ongoing research in the field of FXS is focused on increasing our understanding of the correlation between specific genetic defects and the clinical symptoms displayed in affected persons, on improving the current available symptomatic treatment and on discovering new treatment methods. **(Table 8)**

Table 8: Professionals Who Might be Involved in the Care of a Child with Fragile X Syndrome

- Family Physician
- Pediatrician
- Geneticist
- Genetic Counselor
- Developmental Paediatrician
- Pediatric Subspecialists (neurologist, cardiologist, ear, nose and throat surgeon, ophthalmologist)
- Speech and Language Pathologist
- Occupational Therapist
- Physiotherapist
- Psychologist
- Special Education Teacher
- Social Worker
- Others

Resources

Fragile X Research Foundation of Canada
167 Queen St. West
Brampton, ON, Canada L6Y 1M5
(905) 453-9366
email: FXRFC@ibm.net
www.fragile-x.ca

Fragile X Resource Centre
c/o Ongwanada, Developmental Counseling Service
191 Portsmouth Avenue
Kingston, ON, Canada
(613) 548-4417
Fax: (613) 548-8135

FRAXA Research Foundation, Inc.
45 Pleasant St.
Newburyport, MA 01950 USA
(978) 462-1866
Fax: (978) 463-9985
Email: fraxa@seacoast.com
http://www.fraxa.org

National Fragile X Foundation
P.O. Box 190488
San Francisco, CA 94119 USA
(510) 763-6036, 1-800-688-8765
Fax: (510) 763-6223
Email: natlfx@sprintmail.com
http://www.fragilex.org

Reading List

Dillworth, W. (Ed.). (1998). *Fragile X: A to Z, A Guide for Families*. FRAXA Research Foundation: West Newbury, Mass.

Dykens, E. M., Hodapp, R. M., & Leckman, J. F. (1994). *Behavior and Development in Fragile X Syndrome*. Thousand Oaks, CA: Sage.

Hagerman, R. J. & Hagerman, P. J. (2002). *Fragile X Syndrome: Diagnosis, Treatment and Research, 3rd ed*. Baltimore, MD: Johns Hopkins University Press.

Spiridigliozzi, G., Lachiewicz, A. M., Macmurdo, C. S., Vizoso, A. D., O'Donnell, C. M., McConkie-Rosell, A., et al. (1997). *Educating Boys with Fragile X Syndrome: A Guide for Parents and Professionals*. Durham, NC: Duke University Medical Center.

Tranfaglia, M. R. (2000). *A Medication Guide for Fragile X Syndrome*. West Newbury, MA: FRAXA Research Foundation.

Weber, J.D. (2000). *Children with Fragile X Syndrome: A Parent's Guide*. Bethesda, MD: Woodbine House.

Wilson, P., Stackhouse, T., O'Connor, R., Scharfenaker, S., & Hagerman, R. (1994). *Issues and Strategies for Educating Children with Fragile X Syndrome: A Monograph*. Denver, CO: Spectra and the National Fragile X Foundation.

References

Abeduto, L., & Hagerman, R. J. (1997). Language and communication in Fragile X syndrome. *Mental Retardation and Developmental Disabilities Research Reviews, 3*, 313-322.

American Academy of Pediatrics Committee on Genetics. (1996). Health supervision for children with fragile X syndrome. *Pediatrics, 98*, 297-300.

Bailey, D. B., Hatton, D. D., & Skinner, M. (1998). Early developmental trajectories of males with fragile X syndrome. *American Journal on Mental Retardation, 103,* 29-39.

Baumgardner, T. L., Reiss, A. L., Freund, L. S., & Abrams, M. T. (1995). Specification of the neurobehavioral phenotype in males with fragile X syndrome. *Pediatrics, 95,* 744-752.

Brown, W. T., Nolin, S., Houck, G. Jr., Ding, X., Glicksman, A, Li, S. Y., et al. (1996). Prenatal diagnosis and carrier screening for fragile X by PCR. *American Journal of Medical Genetics, 64,* 191-195.

Butler, M. G., Allen, G. A., Haynes, J. L., Singh, D. N., Watson, M. S., & Breg, W. R. (1991). Anthropometric comparison of mentally retarded males with and without the fragile X syndrome. *American Journal of Medical Genetics, 38,* 260-268.

Davids, J. R., Hagerman, R. J., & Eilert, R. E. (1990). Orthopaedic aspects of fragile X syndrome. *Journal of Bone and Joint Surgery- American, 72,* 889-896.

deVries, B. B., Wiegers, A. M., Smits, A. P., Mohkamsung, S., Duivenvoorden, H. J., Oostra, B. A., et al. (1996). Mental status of females with an FMR1 gene full mutation. *American Journal of Medical Genetics, 58,* 1025-1032.

Feinstein, C., & Reiss, A. L. (1998). Autism: The point of view from fragile X studies. *Journal of Autism and Developmental Disorders, 28,* 393-405.

Friefeld, S., MacGregor, D., & Silverstein, C. (1991). The occupational performance needs of children with fragile X syndrome. *Canadian Journal of Occupational Therapy, 58(Supplement),* 42.

Friefeld, S., Rosenfield, J., Laframboise, K., MacGregor, D., Markovitch, S., Teshima, I., et al. (1993). The Fragile X syndrome: A multidisciplinary perspective on clinical features, diagnosis and intervention. *Journal on Developmental Disabilities, 2,* 56-72.

Franke, P., Leboyer, M., Gansicke, M., Wieffenbach, O., Biancalana, V., Cornillet-Lefebre, P., et al. (1998). Genotype-phenotype relationship in female carriers of the premutation and full mutation of FMR-1. *Psychiatry Research, 80,* 113-127.

Freund, L. S., & Reiss, A. L. (1991). Cognitive profiles associated with the fra(X) syndrome in males and females. *American Journal of Medical Genetics, 38,* 542-547.

Freund, L. S., Reiss, A. L., & Abrams, M. T. 1993). Psychiatric disorders associated with fragile X in the young female. *Pediatrics, 91,* 321-329.

Fu, Y. H., Kuhl, D. P., Pizzuti, A., Piereti, M., Sutcliffe, J. S., Richards, S., et al. (1991). Variation of the CGG repeat at the fragile X site results in genetic instability: resolution of the Sherman Paradox. *Cell, 67,* 1047-1058.

Hagerman, R. J. (1996). Medical follow-up and pharmacotherapy. In R.J. Hagerman, and A. Cronister (Eds.), *Fragile X Syndrome: Diagnosis, Treatment and Research* (2nd ed., pp. 283-331). Baltimore, MD: Johns Hopkins University Press.

Hagerman, R. J. (1999). Fragile X Syndrome. In R.J. Hagerman (Ed.), *Neurodevelopmental Disorders: Diagnosis and Treatment* (pp. 61-132). New York, NY: Oxford University Press.

Hagerman, R. J., Altshul-Stark, D., & McBogg, P. (1987). Recurrent otitis media in the fragile X syndrome. *American Journal of Diseases in Childhood, 141*, 184-187.

Hagerman, R. J., Amiri, K., & Cronister, A. (1991). Fragile X checklist. *American Journal of Medical Genetics, 38*, 283-287.

Hagerman, R. J., Hull, C. E., Safanda, J. F., Carpenter, I., Staley, L. W., O'Connor, R., et al. (1994). High functioning fragile X males: Demonstration of an unmethylated fully expanded FMR-1 mutation associated with protein expression. *American Journal of Medical Genetics, 51*, 298-308.

Hatton, D. D., Buckley, E., Lachiewicz, A., & Roberts, J. (1998). Ocular status of boys with fragile X syndrome: A prospective study. *Journal of AAPOS : the official publication of the American Association for Pediatric Ophthalmology and Strabismus / American Association for Pediatric Ophthalmology and Strabismus, 2*, 298-302.

Hodapp, R., Leckman, J., Dykens, E. M., Sparrow, S. S., Zelinsky, D. G., & Ort, S. I. (1992). K-ABC profiles in children with fragile X syndrome, Down syndrome and non-specific mental retardation. *American Journal on Mental Retardation, 97*, 39-46.

Kaufmann, W. E., Abrams, M. T., Chen, W., & Reiss, A. L. (1999). Genotype, molecular phenotype and cognitive phenotype: Correlations in fragile X syndrome. *American Journal of Human Genetics, 83*, 286-95.

Kaufmann, W. E., & Reiss, A. L. (1999). Molecular and cellular genetics of fragile X syndrome. *American Journal of Medical Genetics, 88*, 11-24.

Kemper, M. B., Hagerman, R. J., & Altshul-Stark, D. (1988). Cognitive profiles of boys with the fragile X syndrome. *American Journal of Medical Genetics, 30*, 191-200.

Lachiewicz, A. M., & Dawson, D. V. (1994). Behavior problems of young girls with fragile X syndrome: Factor scores on the Conners' Parent's Questionnaire. *American Journal of Medical Genetics, 51*, 364-369.

Loesch, D. Z., Huggins, R. M., & Hoang, N. H. (1995). Growth in stature in fragile X families: A mixed longitudinal study. *American Journal of Medical Genetics, 58*, 249-256.

Lubs, H. A. (1969). A marker X chromosome. *American Journal of Human Genetics, 21*, 231-244.

Lubs, H. A., Schwartz, C. E., Stevenson, R. E., & Arena, J. F. (1996). Study of X-linked mental retardation (XLMR): Summary of 61 families in the Miami/Greenwood Study. *American Journal of Medical Genetics, 64,* 169-175.

Martin, J. P., & Bell, J. (1943). A pedigree of mental defect showing sex linkage. *Journal of Neurological Psychiatry, 6,* 154-157.

McCabe, E. R. B., de la Cruz, F., & Clapp, K. (1999). Workshop on fragile X: Future research directions. *American Journal of Medical Genetics, 85,* 317-322.

McConkie-Rosell, A., Robinson, H., Wake, S., Staley, L. W., Heller, K., & Cronister, A. (1995). Dissemination of genetic risk information to relatives in the fragile X syndrome: Guidelines for genetic counselors. *American Journal of Medical Genetics, 59,* 426-430.

Merenstein, S. A., Sobesky, W. E., Taylor, A. K., Riddle, J. E., Tran, H. X., & Hagerman, R. J. (1996). Molecular-clinical correlations in males with an expanded FMR1 mutation. *American Journal of Medical Genetics, 64,* 388-394.

Miller, L. J., McIntosh, D. N., McGrath, J., Shyu, V., Lampe, M., Taylor, A. K., et al. (1999). Electrodermal responses to sensory stimuli in individuals with fragile X syndrome: A preliminary report. *American Journal of Medical Genetics, 83,* 268-279.

Mostofsky, S. H., Mazzocco, M. M., Aakalu, G., Warsofsky, I. S., Denckla, M. B., & Reiss, A. L. (1998). Decreased cerebellar posterior vermis size in fragile X syndrome. *American Academy of Neurology, 50,* 121-130.

Musumeci, S. A., Hagerman, R. J., Ferri, R., Bosco, P., Dalla Bernardina, B., Tassinari, C. A., et al. (1999). Epilepsy and EEG findings in males with fragile X syndrome. *Epilepsia, 40,* 1092-1099.

Nolin, S. L., Lewis, F.A., III., Ye, L. L., Houck, G. E., Jr., Glicksman, A. E., Limprasert, P., et al. (1996). Familial transmission of the FMR1 CGG repeat. *American Journal of Human Genetics, 59,* 1252-1261.

Riddle, J. E., Cheema, A., Sobesky, W. E., Gardner, S. C., Taylor, A. K., Pennington, B. F., et al. (1998). Phenotypic involvement in females with the FMR1 gene mutation. *American Journal on Mental Retardation, 102,* 590-601.

Rousseau, F., Morel, M. L., Rouillard, P., Khandjian, E. W., & Morgan, K. (1996). Surprisingly low prevalence of FMR1 premutation among males of the general population. *American Journal of Human Genetics, 59(suppl),* A188.

Scharfenaker, S., O'Connor, R., Stackhouse, T., Braden, M., Hickman, L., & Gray, K. (1996). An integrated approach to intervention. In R.J. Hagerman & A. Cronister (Eds.), *Fragile X Syndrome: Diagnosis, Treatment and Research* (2nd ed., pp.349-411). Baltimore, MD: Johns Hopkins University Press.

Simko, A., Hornstein, L., Soukup, S., & Bagamery, N. (1989). Fragile X syndrome: Recognition in young children. *Pediatrics, 83,* 547-552.

Sparrow, S.S., Balla, D.A., & Cicchetti, D.V. (1984). *Vineland Adaptive Behavior Scales: Interview edition, Expanded form manual.* Circle Pines, MN: American Guidance Service.

Spiridigliozzi, G., Lachiewicz, A. M., Macmurdo, C. S., Vizoso, A. D., O'Donnell, C. M., McConkie-Rosell, A., et al. (1997). *Educating boys with fragile X syndrome: A guide for parents and professionals.* Durham, NC: Duke University Medical Center.

Staley-Gane, L., Flynn, L., Neitzel, K., Cronister, A., & Hagerman, R. J. (1996). Expanding the role of the genetic counselor. *American Journal of Medical Genetics, 64,* 382-387.

Tassone, F., Hagerman, R. J., Ikle, D., Dyer, P. N., Lampe, M., Willemsen, R., et al. (1999). FMRP production as a potential prognostic indicator in fragile X syndrome. *American Journal of Medical Genetics, 84,* 250-261.

Thorndike, R.L., Hagen, E.P., & Sattler, J.M. (1986). *Guide for administering and scoring the Stanford-Binet Intelligence Scale: Fourth Edition.* Chicago, IL: Riverside.

Turner, G., Webb, T., Wake, S., & Robinson, H. (1996). Prevalence of fragile X syndrome. *American Journal of Medical Genetics, 64,* 196-197.

Verkerk, A. J., Pieretti, M., Sutcliffe, J. S., Fu, Y. H., Kuhl, D. P., Pizzuti, A., et al. (1991). Identification of a gene (FMR-1) containing a CGG repeat coincident with a breakpoint cluster region exhibiting length variation in fragile X syndrome. *Cell, 65,* 905-914.

Vianna-Morgante, A. M. (1999). Twinning and premature ovarian failure in premutation fragile X carriers. *American Journal of Medical Genetics, 83,* 326.

Wilson, P., Stackhouse, T., O'Connor, R., Scharfenaker, S., & Hagerman, R. (1994). *Issues and strategies for educating children with fragile X syndrome: A monograph.* Denver, CO: Spectra and the National Fragile X Foundation.

Wolff, P. H., Gardner, J., Paccia, J., & Lappen, J. (1989). The greeting behavior of fragile X males. *American Journal on Mental Retardation, 93,* 406-411.

Wright-Talamante, C., Cheema, A., Riddle, J. E., Luckey, D. W., Taylor, A. K., & Hagerman, R. J. (1996). A controlled study of longitudinal IQ changes in females and males with fragile X syndrome. *American Journal of Medical Genetics, 64,* 350-355.

York, A., von Fraunhofer, N., Turk, J., & Sedgwick, P. (1999). Fragile-X syndrome, down syndrome and autism: Awareness and knowledge amongst special educators. *Journal of Intellectual Disability Research, 43(Pt 4),* 314-324.

Yu, S., Pritchard, M., Kremer, E., Lynch, M., Nancarrow, J., Baker, E., et al. (1991). Fragile X genotype characterized by and unstable region of DNA. *Science, 252,* 1179-1181.

CHAPTER 3

Down Syndrome

Robert J. Pary

Introduction

Clinicians have been interested in persons with Down syndrome for many years. Pueschel and Pueschel (1992) note that Esquirol described a child with what eventually would be called Down syndrome in 1838. John Langdon Down (1866) provided detail about the physical signs and later Down (1887) provided behavioral characteristics such as stubbornness and self-talk. Down (1866) contrasted persons with the syndrome he called "mongolism" from those with "cretinism" (congenital hypothyroidism).

Often, it is hard for families, friends and clinicians to read about the history of this syndrome and realize that the initial descriptions referred to "mongoloids" or "mongoloid idiots". Even in the mid-20th century, Jervis (1948) wrote about "mongoloid idiocy" in a classic paper about dementia in persons with Down syndrome. Consequently, as an antidote to these pejorative terms and stereotypes, this chapter will liberally use quotes from an excellent book written by two persons with Down syndrome.

> *I'm glad to have Down syndrome. I think it's a good thing to have for all people that are born with it. I don't think it's a handicap. It's a disability*

for what you're learning because you're learning slowly. It's not that bad.

There's a lot of things I did a lot of other people don't do. Like being in two different shows, going to a lot of conventions, award ceremonies like the Kennedy's, and I'm a famous actor. First of all, when I was three, that's when I started to be in the show 'This is My Son' . . . When I was three through sixteen I was filming 'Sesame Street'.

Six years before, when I was ten, I filmed "The Fall Guy." I got to learn a sixty-four-page script. How can a Down syndrome kid memorize a sixty-four-page script? But I did it. In "The Fall Guy" I acted with Lee Majors . . . I am teaching Lee Majors how to count in three foreign languages: Spanish, French and Japanese. *(Kingsley & Levitz, 1994, p. 35-36).*

Jason's quote probably is not the typical picture that most people have when they think of someone with Down syndrome. This chapter is about what people with Down syndrome can teach us as well as what is known about Down syndrome.

One of the things that people with Down syndrome can teach us is that some of their hopes and aspirations are similar to most people's dreams. The following excerpt is from an article where the lead author is a person with Down Syndrome. Mike talks about his desire for a better job and what he would like about his new job.

My name is Michael Paul Lauris. I am 35-years-old. I work at the Pittsburgh Blind Association and have worked there for eight years. I would like to move on to a better paying job, near where I live. I would like to work in a grocery store as a bagger because I would be able to meet and talk with people. I would like to help them with their groceries and ask them how they are doing. . . I have applied for a job at Foodland near where I live, and I will find out soon if I got the job. (Lauris & Pary, 1993, p. 62).

As one reads the information about biomedical features, psychological features and vulnerabilities and social features and vulnerabilities, it is important not to forget two images. One is ten-year-old Jason Kinglsey memorizing a 64-page script and teaching his cast member how to count in Japanese. The second image is that of Mike Lauris applying for a job at Foodland because it will offer better pay, be close to where he lives, and let him have more social interactions.

Biomedical Features

Cause of Down syndrome

Down syndrome is one of the most common types of genetic disorders. Approximately one child in eight hundred live births will have Down syndrome. The characteristics of Down syndrome result from an extra copy of chromosome 21. The extra copy occurs because of dysfunction during cell division.

There are three kinds of genetic variations leading to extra chromosome material. The most common (about 95%) chromosomal variation in Down syndrome is trisomy 21. This refers to having three copies instead of two of chromosome 21. Although the vast majority of persons with Down syndrome have three copies of chromosome 21, technically, <u>not</u> everyone with Down syndrome has trisomy 21. Instead of trisomy 21, some people have either translocation or mosaicism.

Translocation means that the extra chromosome 21 splits apart and attaches to another chromosome. The other chromosome may be 21, but it can also be 14 or 22. Translocation occurs about 3-4%. The rarest chromosomal variation is mosaicism. This means that not all of the person's cells show an extra chromosome 21. Mosaicism happens in 1-2% of persons with Down syndrome.

The Diagnosis of Down Syndrome

The diagnosis of Down syndrome can be made while the mother is still pregnant. The fetus' cells taken from amniotic fluid or placenta are tested. The fetus' cells will show if there is extra chromosome 21 material. Murray and Cohen counsel prospective parents of a newborn with Down syndrome to talk about their feelings and their fears about having a child Down syndrome. The following is an excerpt from *Count Us In* when Mitchell Levitz, who has Down syndrome, asks about his father's reaction.

> *Mitchell:* I am quite interested in knowing what your feelings are about me when I was born with Down syndrome.
>
> *Jack:* Well, the interesting thing was, that you probably don't know about, when Mommy was student-teaching during college, teaching special ed, there were a few kids in her class with Down syndrome. They had class trips and I used to go with her and we used to talk.
>
> When you're getting married, you talk about your plans, and we had said that sometimes after we had our regular family we'd like to adopt a child with Down syndrome. When you were born, the news was devastating. I thought I wouldn't have anyone to help me cut the grass or shovel the snow. And since you were my first son, I immediately thought about the Bar Mitzvah and I thought you wouldn't be able to have a Bar Mitzvah. So, even though I had once wanted to adopt a child with Down syndrome, I didn't expect you to be born with Down syndrome. So that was my reaction. (Kingsley & Levitz, 1994, p. 37).

Mitchell reacts puzzledly. He cannot understand why his dad would want to adopt someone with Down syndrome, before his dad knew that Mitchell would come into his dad's life. This vignette captures that not only do parents have complicated feelings about their children being born with Down syndrome, but also some persons with Down syndrome wonder what his or her parents felt at the birth.

The Diagnostic Features of Down Syndrome

The most common features in children with Down syndrome include a) flattened face with a low nasal bridge and a small nose; b) upward slant to the eyes; c) skin folds in the inner aspects of the eyes; d) floppy muscle tone e) increased mobility of the joints; f) a small or undeveloped middle bone of the fifth finger; g) single crease across the center of the palm; h) abnormal position and/or shape of the ear; I) Brushfield spots (a ring of white spots in the iris' periphery); j) lack of a Moro reflex (when a baby is startled, the Moro reflex is for the arms to go up and away from the body.).

Pueschel (1992) notes several physical features of Down syndrome. The mouth may have one or more distinctive features such as an open mouth, protruding tongue, high-arched palate, narrow palate, and abnormal teeth. The tongue may appear to be enlarged in relationship to the small mouth. The neck can be short. The movement of the neck is supple unless there is symptomatic atlantoaxial dislocation (neck pain or evidence of spinal cord injury). The Pueschels note that congenital heart defects have been reported in between 19% to 55% in surveys of physical features of persons with Down syndrome. Other extremity features include short, broad hands, in-curved fifth finger, and a gap between the first and second toes. Short stature is another common feature.

The Pueschels discuss that the physical features of Down syndrome change over time. Epicanthal folds may become less obvious. Others, such as a fissured tongue or looking older that the chronological age, do not occur until later in life. Some features like the flattened back of the head or single palmar crease remain throughout life.

Diagnostic Test and Genetic Counseling

The genetic mystery of Down syndrome was uncovered in 1959 by Lejeune. The diagnosis of Down syndrome can be done prenatally by sampling amniotic fluid, chorionic villus sampling or percutaneous umbilical blood sampling. Sometimes the diagnosis is not made before birth. In that case, karotyping is recommended to confirm the diagnosis of extra chromosome 21 material. Determining the chromosomal basis for the person having Down syndrome can assist the parents in assessing the odds of having another child with Down syndrome. Although having one child with Down syndrome increases the likelihood of having other children with Down syndrome, in most situations, the risk is only 1-2%. The exception is in the 3-4% of individuals whose Down syndrome resulting from translocation. When the mother is the carrier, the odds increase to 5-10%. If the translocation, however, is 21/21, then the odds are 100%.

The other reason to check a person's chromosomes is for persons who have been diagnosed with Down syndrome, but who do not have a typical presentation (a middle-aged adult who looks *younger* than his/her stated age). As will be discussed below, people with Down syndrome have different risks for certain illnesses (e.g., dementia or bipolar disease) than do persons in the general population. Misdiagnosing someone with Down syndrome may make family or clinicians much more concerned about dementia than would be warranted.

Medical Risks

There is a lot of information about routine medical screening for persons with Down syndrome. Unfortunately, persons with Down syndrome are at increased risk for a number of conditions (e.g. hypothyroidism). As a guide to families and caregivers, the American Academy of Pediatrics (2001) and Cohen (1999) have published guidelines for schedule of routine supervision. Lott and McCoy (1992) advocate a screening schedule. The following has been adapted from their recommendations as well as Van Allen, Fung, and Jurenka (1999).

Neonate and Infancy
1) Check the eyes for the red reflex. This is a screen for cataracts.
2) Observe for vomiting and/or the absence of stools. Some infants with Down syndrome are born with a blockage of the gastrointestinal system.
3) Check for blue, dusky color of the skin (cyanosis). Feel the pulse and/or apical heart beat for an irregular rhythm. Listen to the heart for murmurs. Check EKG. Consider an echocardiogram. These are screens for congenital heart disease.
4) Check thyroid function tests for signs of thyroid disease.
5) Do a hearing screen (auditory brain stem evoked response).
6) Consider referral to a parent's support group.
7) Consider referral to an early intervention program.

Pre-School (1-5 years)
1) Screen for orthopedic problems (e.g., dislocated hips).
2) Consider screen for atlanto-axial dislocation.
3) Perform dental exam.
4) Do ENT exam with microscopic otoscopy if ear canals do not permit routine pediatric exam.
5) Complete ophthalmologic exam.
6) Do annual thyroid testing.
7) Perform vaccination schedule including influenzal, pneumoccal, and hepatitis B vaccines for children at major risk.
8) Obtain speech and language assessment.
9) Consider developmental assessments (physical, occupational, and feeding/nutritional).
10) Continue early intervention programs.

Elementary and High School Years
1) Consider doing a cervical spine x-ray.
2) Do annual dental exam.
3) Perform annual audiogram.
4) Do annual ophthalmological exam.

5) Check thyroid function annually.
6) Provide nutritional and dietary consultation as needed.
7) Start an individualized exercise program modified for any orthopedic or other health reasons. Provide guidance regarding participation in sports.
8) Continue speech and language programs as needed.
9) Do psycho-educational evaluation every three years.
10) Consider vocational training/supervised work programs.
11) Begin to develop skills for independent living and separation from family.
12) Monitor for sleep problems such as snoring or apneic spells. Consider a sleep study if obstructive sleep apnea is suspected.

Adulthood (18-50 years)
1) Consider doing a cervical spine x-ray.
2) Do annual dental exam.
3) Consider counseling if transition from school to workplace becomes difficult. Consider counseling to assist in separation from family and to assist in independent living if this is a reasonable goal.
4) Do regular ophthalmological and audiological exam.
5) Check thyroid function annually.
6) Provide nutritional and dietary consultation as needed.
7) Continue an individualized exercise program modified for any orthopedic or other health reasons.
8) Consider annual complete blood count (CBC), urinalysis, renal function tests and lipid profile.
9) Regular pelvic exam and Pap smear (frequency depends on risks of disease).
10) Chest X-ray when history and/or physical exam are suggested of pneumonia.
11) Monitor for seizures.
12) Monitor for major depression. Observe for sleep disturbance, eating disturbance, low energy, low mood, etc.
13) Monitor for unresolved grief reactions.
14) Check for snoring and/or apneic spells. Consider referral for sleep studies.

Elderly Persons (50+ years)
1) Continue all adult screens that are appropriate (e.g. counseling for transition from school to work is not relevant).
2) Screen for osteoporosis.
3) Monitor for gait deterioration.
4) Monitor for functional decline. This includes loss of activity of daily living skills and cognitive decline. If functional decline is present, search for reversible causes (e.g. hypothyroidism). If reversible causes are not present, consider evaluation for Alzheimer disease.
5) Pay attention to development of cataracts.
6) Monitor for possibility of gastroesophageal reflux disease.
7) Check for genitourinary problems. These disorders include recurrent urinary tract infections and bladder resection.

Psychological Features

Is there a psychological and behavioral pheneotype in persons with Down syndrome?

A behavioral phenotype is a pattern of particular cognitive, motor, speech, and social ways that are consistently associated with a genetic disorder. Udwin and Dennis (1995) reviewed the evidence for a psychological and behavioral phenotype in persons with Down syndrome.

They concluded that in Down syndrome IQs center around 55 (instead of 100 in the general population). Only ten percent of persons with Down syndrome have IQs in the "normal" range. Ninety percent have IQs in the range of mental retardation or borderline intellectual functioning. IQs tend to decline as children with Down syndrome age. Furthermore, there is a general slowing of thinking. Yet it appears that the authors of *Count Us In*, Jason Kingsley and Mitchell Levitz, who both have Down syndrome, stand in stark contrast to this picture of a decline of IQ. At this stage, it is not known whether the authors are very unique or whether the rich environment and high expectations they have for themselves have made the difference.

Another common trait that Udwin and Dennis (1995) mention regarding a behavioral phenotype in persons with Down syndrome is problems in speaking. Generally, people with Down syndrome understand more and have a greater desire to communicate, than they can actually enunciate. Jason and Mitchell discuss speaking. The stimulus is a discussion that ensues after Jason mentions that he wants to become a teacher's aide so that he can teach kids.

> *Mitchell: . . . From my experience, people have a hard time understanding me because of my speech.*
>
> *Jason: I have the best speech in the world . . . I don't think people can't understand what I'm saying. I have a very good speech. I get speech therapy.*
>
> *Mitchell: From my point of view, the important thing is not that they don't understand you, it could help you project, help you speak better. Then, in the future more people could understand you much better if you have good fluency in order to express yourself. Like for example, if I were going to have an interview for college, I should speak more clear so they could understand the information I'd tell them so they could know ... what kind of reason I have . . . (Kingsley & Levitz, 1994).*

In the 1800's, John Langdon Down contributed to the quest for a behavioral phenotype when he noted that persons with the syndrome subsequently named after him were humorous, stubborn, tended to imitate, and talked to themselves.

Psychiatric or Behavioral Risks

Autism

Autism is a disorder beginning before three years of age. It consists of problems in communication, social interactions, symbolic or imaginative play and repetitive behavior. The lack of social imitative play may be a clue that a child with Down syndrome may also have autism. Back in the 1800's, Down noted that mimicry was a central feature of persons with Down syndrome. The association between autism and Down syndrome is unclear. Pary (1993) reviewed studies that provided percentages of autism in clinic populations. The studies were from the United States (Myers & Pueschel, 1991), England (Collacott, Cooper, & McGrother, 1992) and Sweden (Lund, 1988). The percentages were 2/235 (0.8%), 8/371 (2.2%) and 5/44 (11%).

Major Depressive Disorder

Nearly everyone has felt sad at one time. Major depressive disorder is diagnosed only when the sadness lasts for at least two weeks and is accompanied by problems with eating, sleeping, concentrating, and feeling fatigued. Suicidal ideation can occur as can feelings of excessive guilt. There is the suspicion that persons with Down syndrome suffer from major depression more often than do others. There are numerous case reports and small studies of people with Down syndrome who suffered from severe depression. Some were suffering so much that electroconvulsive therapy was needed because medications did not work and the person was eating so little that their life was in danger.

In the review by Pary (1993) noted above, the studies from the United States, England and Sweden revealed percentages of depression of 6%, 11%, and 0%, respectively. The 6% drops to 4% in the US study, if one includes persons with Down syndrome who were living in an institution. Pary, Strauss, and White (1996) did a population survey of major depression in over 11,000 persons with Down syndrome in California. Contrary to expectations, major depression was recognized and diagnosed significantly less often than in persons with other etiologies for mental retardation.

Treatment generally includes an antidepressant medication. Sometimes, treatment can include psychotherapy, with modifications to process to accommodate for expressive language deficits. If there are psychotic symptoms, a neuroleptic may be prescribed. Rarely, electroconvulsive therapy will need to be considered when the symptoms reach a stage of life-threatening (Warren, Holroyd, & Folstein, 1989).

Bipolar Disorder

Bipolar disorder is the current term for manic depression. A person suffers from serious highs and lows in mood. Symptoms of mania may include demonstrating excessive energy, requiring less sleep, speaking and thinking much faster, having a greater drive for sexual activity such as compulsively masturbating, and believing that he or she possesses special powers. The mood can be always joking and in excessively good spirits or there can be constant irritability. Pary, Strauss, and White

(1996) also looked at bipolar illness in the survey of over 11,000 persons with Down syndrome in California. They did not find any persons diagnosed with bipolar illness.

Pary, Friedlander, and Capone (1999) reviewed their clinical records and found six persons with Down syndrome and suspected bipolar disorder. Those increased the number of persons known to have bipolar disorder and Down syndrome to only 15 in publications in English. This is far, far less than would be predicted based upon the prevalence of Bipolar Disorder in the general population.

In the few cases of persons with Down syndrome and Bipolar Disorder, a mood stabilizer such as lithium, carbamazepine, or valproic acid would be prescribed.

Psychosis

Psychosis can be difficult to diagnose in persons with IQs under 45. As with other psychiatric disorders and Down syndrome, this is another area of some controversy. Over a hundred years ago, Down noted that persons with Down syndrome tended to talk to themselves. Sovner and Hurley (1993) have cautioned that self-talk is not necessarily a sign of psychosis. Overall, it appears that schizophrenia is less common in persons with Down syndrome. In clinical experience, there are some people with Down syndrome who have a major depression and also have psychotic features. In some cases, a neuroleptic medication to treat the psychotic part of the illness will also be needed.

Obsessive Compulsive Disorder

In the 1800s, John Langdon Down noted that persons with the syndrome bearing his name tended to be obstinate. Sometimes this stubbornness can reach to the degree of obsessional slowness (Pary, 1994). These are persons who take an extremely long time to do activity of daily living skills (bathing and dressing). Eating a meal can take hours. Obsessive Compulsive Disorder can be difficult to treat. Obsessive slowness may respond to "pacing," that is, using a clock and setting the time to complete a task. Pacing seems simple but it can be difficult to operationalize. Pacing may well worsen symptoms initially.

Medications, such as selective serotonin reuptake inhibitors, are often tried in Obsessive Compulsive Disorder. The results have been modest and sometimes the medication needs to be augmented with another psychotropic medication.

Dementia

Dementia refers to memory decline associated with other cognitive features such as forgetting how to do skills previously mastered (e.g., getting appropriately dressed). The observation that persons with Down syndrome are at risk for developing dementia goes back to the 1800s, not long after the syndrome was described by John Langdon Down. In the first part of the 20th century, life expectance for persons with Down syndrome seldom reached adulthood. Individuals with Down syndrome seldom lived long enough to get dementia. However, by the mid-20th century, health care had improved and persons with Down syndrome were living longer. As they lived into their 50s and 60s, clinicians and families observed that a number of adults showed a functional decline. By 1948, Jervis concluded that persons with Down syndrome may be at increased risk for developing dementia.

Individuals with Alzheimer disease in the general population have characteristic changes in their brains. These changes include beta-amyloid plaques, neurofibrillary tangles and neuronal loss. Similar findings can be seen in almost all postmortem brains of persons with Down syndrome who are older than 40 years old. Nevertheless, not everyone with Down syndrome older than 40 years have dementia. Estimates of dementia in adults with Down syndrome range from 15 to 51% (Lott, 2002). The average age of developing dementia is in the early 50s.

Evenhuis (1990) described the natural history of dementia in persons with Down syndrome. Interestingly, she found that the onset of dementia did not significantly differ between persons with Down syndrome and either moderate or more severe mental retardation. Both groups had an onset of dementia in the early 50s. Furthermore, the duration of the symptoms of dementia until death did not seem significantly different. Death occurred about five years after the onset of symptoms.

Evenhuis, however, concluded that the early symptoms of dementia are different depending upon whether the person has moderate or severe mental retardation. The hallmark of dementia is a decline in recent memory. Unfortunately, Evenhuis found, that in persons with severe mental retardation, memory or spatial/temporal orientation could not be assessed. In persons with Down syndrome and more severe mental retardation, the keys to the diagnosis of dementia are the early symptoms of apathy, withdrawal, and a decline in activity of daily living skills, seizures, and gait deterioration.

In distinction, Evenhuis noted that in persons with moderate mental retardation and Down syndrome, dementia could be screened for with tests of short-term memory and orientation. Only a third of her sample (3/9) showed recent memory decline in the first year. Even fewer showed disorientation. By the third year, all nine demonstrated impairment in orientation and recent memory. The most common symptom in the early stages of both the severe and the moderate group were apathy and withdrawal. The association between dementia and depression is complex. Major depression is considered as one of the differential diagnoses to rule out when a person has a functional decline. Burt, Loveland, and Lewis (1992) cataloged the symptoms common to both Alzheimer disease and major depression in persons with Down syndrome. These include apathy, loss of self-help skills, depression, urinary incontinence, psychomotor slowing, uncooperativeness, loss of housekeeping skills, greater dependency, loss of interest in surroundings, weight loss, and sleep problems. When in doubt between major depression and dementia, some clinicians will often treat with an antidepressant because major depression is reversible with treatment and dementia cannot be cured.

The management of someone with dementia and Down syndrome includes paying attention to safety issues such as wandering, providing assistance in activities of daily living, and determining when a nursing home is needed as in persons with dementia in the general population. Drug treatment involves slowing the progression of the dementia. There is no cure for dementia and the illness probably can not be reversed.

Strategies include vitamin E and anticholinesterase medications such as donepezil, galantamine and rivastigmine. There is relatively little information about treatment. There are two recent studies of donepezil in persons with Down syndrome (Lott, Osann, Doran, & Nelson, 2002; Prasher, Huxley, & Haque, 2002). Prasher's group found that 50% of the donepezil group (8 out of 16 persons) and 20% of the placebo (sugar pill) group had serious side effects. These side effects were diarrhea, insomnia, fatigue and nausea. Furthermore, Prasher's group did not find a statistically significant result, though the sample size was small. Nevertheless, they concluded that donepezil was safe and merits further study. Lott's group was a pilot study and found that donepezil may be helpful and also emphasized that further study is needed.

Other Behavioral Concerns

Although there are individuals with aggression, self-injury, and other maladaptive behaviors, the question often is whether this is a nonspecific function of having a developmental disability or are these behaviors more common in Down syndrome? Dykens and Kasari (1997) looked at the maladaptive behavior in children with Down syndrome, Prader-Willi syndrome, and nonspecific etiologies of mental retardation. They found that children with Down syndrome had less maladaptive behaviors than persons with Prader-Willi syndrome. Interestingly, obsessions were similar to persons with nonspecific etiologies and significantly less than children with Prader-Willi syndrome. Furthermore, compulsive behavior was significantly less in those with Down syndrome compared to children with Prader-Willi syndrome. There was no behavior that separated children with Down syndrome from the other two groups. There were only a few features that were significantly different between boys and girls with Down syndrome and those with nonspecific etiologies of mental retardation. Children with Down syndrome were significantly more likely to have speech problems and to prefer being alone.They were similar in these regards to children with Prader-Willi syndrome. Children with nonspecific etiologies of mental retardation were significantly more likely to be hyperactive than either of the other two groups. There was no maladaptive behavior that was more common in children with Down syndrome than those with Prader-Willi syndrome.

Common Myths

Udwin and Dennis (1995) mention that many people think of children with Down syndrome as generally amiable. While this is often true, up to a fourth of infants can be quite difficult to engage and some could qualify for a disorder of conduct in adolescence.

Social Features and Vulnerabilities

Educational Opportunities

One of the most surprising parts of the *Count Us In* is in the chapter on "Our Future Plans." Jason is concerned that his friend Mitchell is rushing through his preparation for his career.

> *Jason: . . . In my opinion . . . I don't think he (Mitchell) should skip College. There's lots of things he might learn because a college prepares him for his future.He does not go anywhere if he skips college. He goes into an apartment with his friends to prepare him for the future. What I'm saying is that there is a big gap right before Jespy and his senior year of high school . . . I advise him that he should go back to college.*
>
> *Emily (Kingsley): Well, he did almost two years at Jespy and now he's going to move into his own place and he's starting a good job at the Peekskill/*
>
> *Corlandt Chamber of Commerce. He'll be working as an office assistant, answering phones, helping to give out information to walk-in customers, filing, faxing, and working on database computer projects. So he seems to bedoing okay.*
>
> *Jason: What I'm saying is, he's getting his low-paying job at the Chamber of Commerce. To make a high-paying job is getting the skills what you need at college right before Jespy so he would have more feedback to his future. I'm really worried about Mitchell's future and his success because he doesn't go anywhere and it doesn't make sense that he skips college . . .*
>
> *Both of us want to have good high-paying jobs and a good future.* (Kingsley & Levitz, 1994, p. 178)

Sociosexual Development

Mike Lauris who has Down syndrome and was 35 years when this was written talks about his best friend.

> *.... I have a roommate, who is also my best friend. His name is Ron, and I have known him for 20 years. We have been living together for about two and one half years. We share the cleaning, cooking and grocery shopping. We watch and share videos. We both like to watch football, baseball, soccer, hockey and basketball and video wrestling tapes and listen to the oldies on the stereo. I met Ron when I was 15-years-old at the school we both went to. He was throwing a baseball and hit me in the nose. Ron and the coach came over to check my nose and it was okay. Ron and I were buddies after that.*

Mike also talks about his goals in his final paragraph.

> *I have accomplished a lot of things in my life and I am working very on losing weight. I have lost eleven pounds over the past five months. I would like to keep going the I am with losing weight. I'm going to lose this crummy belly of mine. I feel happy; life is WOW! Exciting. The most important thing I want is to keep putting one foot ahead of the other. One last thing I want to put in this paper is I want marriage in my life.* (Lauris & Pary, 1993).

Jason and Mitchell also talk about marriage. Both want to get married and have children. Mitchell talks about adopting a child, if he and his future wife could not have one by themselves. There is a need for education on sexuality. A British study found that young people with Down syndrome were inadequately prepared to consider their sexuality, including sexual relationships (Shepperdson, 1995). A recent review of medical care for adolescents with Down syndrome also emphasizes that sexuality, as well as issue of sexual abuse, pregnancy and menstrual hygiene need to be openly discussed (Rozien, 2002)

Common Myths

The myth is that persons with Down syndrome are asexual and have little interest in sex or relationships. The above section clearly disputes this myth.

Summary

This chapter has attempted to shatter some of the stereotypes about persons with Down syndrome. While there are certain medical and psychiatric concerns, the words of people with Down syndrome suggest that their dreams are not much different than the rest of us.

References

American Academy of Pediatrics. (2001). Health supervision for children with Down syndrome. *Pediatrics, 107*, 442-449.

Burt, D. B., Loveland, K. A., & Lewis, K. R. (1992). Depression and the onset of dementia in adults with mental retardation. *American Journal on Mental Retardation, 96*, 502-511.

Cohen, W. I. (1999, Sept.). Health care guidelines for individuals with Down syndrome. *Down Syndrome Quarterly, 4.*

Collacott, R. A., Cooper, S. A., & McGrother, C. (1992). Differential rates of psychiatricdisorders in adults with Down's syndrome compared with other mentally retarded adults. *British Journal of Psychiatry, 161*, 671-674.

Down, J. L. (1866). Observation of an ethnic classification of idiots. *London Hospital: Clinical Lectures and Report, 3*, 259-262.

Down, J. L. (1887). *Mental Affections of Childhood and Youth* (reprinted as *Classics in Developmental Medicine* (No. 5) (1990). London: MacKeith Press.

Dykens, E. M, & Kasari, C. (1997). Maladaptive behavior in children with Prader-Willi syndrome, Down syndrome, and nonspecific mental retardation. *American Journal on Mental Retardation, 102,* 228-237.

Evenhuis, H. M. (1990). The natural history of dementia in Down's syndrome. *Archives of Neurology, 47,* 263-267.

Jervis, G. (1948). Early senile dementia in mongoloid idiocy. *American Journal of Psychiatry, 105,* 102-106.

Kingsley, J., & Levitz, M. (1994). *Count Us In.* Orlando, FL: Harcourt Brace.

Lauris, M. P, & Pary, R. J. (1993). Life beyond a psychiatric disorder. *Habilitative Mental Health Newsletter, 12,* 62-63.

Lott, I. T. (2002). Down syndrome and Alzheimer disease. In R. J. Pary (Ed.), *Psychiatric Problems in Older Persons with Developmental Disabilities.* (pp. 25-34). Kingston, NY: NADD Press

Lott, I. T., & McCoy, E. (1992). *Down Syndrome Advances in Medical Care.* New York, NY: Wiley-Liss.

Lott, I. T., Osann, K., Doran, E., & Nelson, L. (2002). Down syndrome and Alzheimer disease: Response to donepezil. *Archives of Neurology, 59,* 1133-1136.

Lund, J. (1988). Psychiatric aspects of Down's syndrome. *Acta psychiatrica Scandinavica, I78,* 369-374.

Murray, N., & Cohen, W. *When your baby has Down syndrome.* Pittsburgh, PA: The Down Syndrome Center, Children's Hospital of Pittsburgh.

Myers, B. A., & Pueschel, S. M. (1991). Psychiatric disorders in persons with Down syndrome. *Journal of Nervous and Mental Disease, 179,* 609-613.

Pary, R. J. (1993). Psychiatric disorders in adults with Down syndrome. *Habilitative Mental Health Newsletter, 12,* 26-27.

Pary, R. J. (1994). Obsessional slowness. *Habilitative Mental Health Newsletter, 13,* 49-50.

Pary, R.J., Friedlander, R., & Capone, G. T. (1999). Bipolar disorder and Down syndrome: Six cases. *Mental Health Aspects of Developmental Disabilities, 2,* 59-63.

Pary, R. J., Strauss, D. J., & White, J. F. (1996). A population survey of bipolar disorder in persons with and without Down syndrome. *Down Syndrome Quarterly, 1(3),* 1-4.

Prasher, V. P., Huxley, A., & Haque, M. S. (2002). A 24-week, double-blind, placebo-controlled trial of donepezil in patients with Down syndrome and Alzheimer's disease: Pilot study. *International Journal of Geriatric Psychiatry, 17,* 270-278.

Pueschel, S., & Pueschel, J. (1992). *Biomedical Concerns in Persons with Down Syndrome.* Baltimore, MD: Paul H. Brookes Publishing Co.

Rozien, N. J. (2002). Medical care and monitoring for the adolescent with Down syndrome. *Adolescent Medicine, 13,* 345-358.

Shepperdson, B. (1995). The control of sexuality in young people with down's syndrome. *Child Care Health Development, 21,* 333-349.

Sovner, R. & Hurley, A. D. (1993). "Psychotoform" psychopathology. *Habilitative Mental Health Newsletter, 12,* 112-113.

Udwin, O., & Dennis, J. (1995). Down syndrome. In G. O'Brien & W. Yule (Eds.), *Behavioural Phenotypes* (pp. 105-109). Cambridge, England: MacKeith Press.

Van Allen, J. I., Fung, J., & Jurenka, S. B. (1999). Health care concerns and guidelines for adults with Down syndrome. *American Journal of Medical Genetics, 89,* 100-110.

Warren, A. C., Holroyd, S., & Folstein, M. F. (1989). Major depression in Down's syndrome. *British Journal of Psychiatry, 155,* 202-205.

CHAPTER 4

Williams Syndrome

Brenda Finucane

Introduction

Williams syndrome has fascinated geneticists and behaviorists for decades, and it is among the most well-researched of the genetic mental retardation syndromes. The condition is associated with an unusual combination of cognitive strengths and weaknesses, as well as a distinctive behavioral phenotype. Co-morbid psychiatric symptoms, particularly attentional disorders, anxiety, and phobias, are common among children and adults with Williams syndrome. The discovery of a specific genetic abnormality linked to Williams syndrome has led to more accurate diagnosis and an increase in research on the molecular correlations with the clinical phenotype.

Williams syndrome is generally estimated to occur 1 in 20,000 births, although a recent Norwegian survey suggests a higher prevalence (Stromme, Bjornstad, & Ramstad, 2002). Most individuals with the disorder fall within the 1% of the population having mental retardation, and its incidence among children and adults with developmental disabilities is approximately 1 in 200. Williams syndrome is thought to account for 6% of those with diagnosed genetic mental retardation syndromes. Professionals working with special needs populations, including those with dual diagnosis, are therefore likely to encounter at least a few people with Williams syndrome over the course of their careers.

Recent interest in Williams syndrome in the popular press and on television has proven to be a double-edged sword. On the positive side, increased public awareness of Williams syndrome has resulted in the diagnosis of many more children and adults with the condition. This not only benefits families, but as the number of those diagnosed grows, researchers gain a clearer understanding of the condition across the full range of age and severity. Unfortunately, some of the unique characteristics of Williams syndrome have been exaggerated in the media, and a stereotypical perception has emerged implying that all people with Williams syndrome show extraordinary musical and linguistic talents. While these appear to be areas of relative strength for people with Williams syndrome, affected individuals show a wide range of abilities, and most do not exhibit unusual linguistic and/or musical talents when compared to typically developing individuals.

Clinical and Laboratory Diagnosis

Williams syndrome was first described as a clinical entity in 1961 by Charles Williams, a physician in New Zealand (Williams, Barrett-Boyes, & Lowe, 1961). The condition is sometimes referred to as Williams-Beuren syndrome because it was almost simultaneously described in the medical literature by a German team (Beuren, Apitz, & Harmjanz, 1962). These initial reports focused on the cute and attractive facial appearance (Figure 1.) seen in affected children, and for several years, the disorder was referred to as the "pixie" or "elfin facies" syndrome, until it was more appropriately renamed Williams syndrome in the 1980's. In Europe, Williams syndrome has also been called the Infantile Hypercalcemia syndrome because of its association with elevated calcium in the blood of some affected infants.

The clinical characteristics of Williams syndrome, particularly the facial appearance, are well-described. Until 1993, when the underlying genetic basis for Williams syndrome was discovered (Ewart et al., 1993), the diagnosis was reliably made by geneticists based on known clinical criteria (Preus, 1984). Laboratory testing is now available which allows objective confirmation of the Williams syndrome diagnosis. Over 99% of people with a clinical diagnosis of Williams syndrome have a microdeletion (submicroscopic missing segment) of the chromosomal locus 7q11. This microdeletion cannot be visualized on standard chromosome testing but can be detected using a molecular FISH probe which is commercially available. Laboratory testing is recommended for all children and adults meeting clinical criteria for Williams syndrome, particularly those with characteristic cardiovascular findings (Committee on Genetics, 2001). Prenatal testing for Williams syndrome is also available, but since the majority of cases occur sporadically with no known familial or environmental risk factors, the diagnosis is rarely made before birth. Babies with Williams syndrome are almost always born to unaffected parents whose chance of having a second child with the disorder is not increased over that of couples in the general population. However, individuals with Williams syndrome have a 50% chance of passing the condition to their offspring. In the past, few adults with Williams syndrome had children, but as opportunities for socialization and independence for people with developmental disabilities increase, familial cases of Williams syndrome (Morris, Thomas, & Greenberg, 1993) are likely to become more common.

The deleted chromosomal region in people with Williams syndrome contains more than a dozen genes, only one of which has been clearly linked to the clinical phenotype. That gene, referred to as ELN, codes for the protein elastin which plays a role in connective tissue elasticity. Some of the syndrome's major findings, including cardiovascular anomalies, joint laxity, and abnormalities of the walls of the bladder and bowel, can potentially be explained by deletion of ELN on one of the two number 7 chromosomes in people with Williams syndrome. Another gene in the 7q11 region, known as the LIM-kinase (or LIMK1) gene, codes for a protein known to be expressed in brain tissue. Researchers have speculated about the role of LIMK1 in producing the characteristic learning profile seen in people with Williams syndrome (Frangiskakis et al., 1996), although the importance of this gene for the neurocognitive phenotype remains unclear (Wu et al., 1998). Ongoing research efforts are aimed at characterizing the remaining genes within the deleted chromosomal region and identifying molecular correlations with the clinical phenotype, particularly the cognitive and behavioral manifestations of Williams syndrome.

Physical Findings and Medical Issues

The facial characteristics of people with Williams syndrome are distinctive and easily recognized in most cases by clinicians familiar with the disorder (Figure 1). The facial appearance in young children and infants is characterized by full lips, puffy cheeks, a relatively long philtrum, and a small jaw. In adolescents and adults, the loss of subcutaneous fat gives the face a more elongated appearance. The eyes often show a starburst ("stellate") pattern in the iris, which is particularly noticeable in blue or light-colored eyes. Many individuals with Williams syndrome have a characteristic raspy, hoarse voice. Short stature is typical, and both children and adults may exhibit joint contractures, sloping shoulders, spinal curvature, and/or a slumped posture.

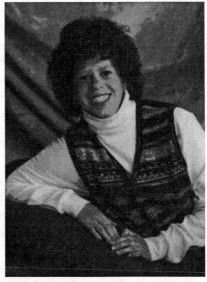

Figure 1
photo courtesy of the Williams Syndrome Association

Sensory impairments are common among children and adults with Williams syndrome. Almost two thirds of those affected develop esotropia (inward deviation of the eye) (Kapp, von Noorden, & Jenkins, 1995), sometimes requiring surgery. Hyperopia (far-sightedness), possibly related to ocular elastin abnormalities, is common and may severely affect vision. Chronic ear infections compound language delays in many young children with Williams syndrome, although these tend to occur less frequently with age. Hyperacusis, or increased sensitivity to sound, is an unusual feature of Williams syndrome found in over 90% of those affected (Klein, Armstrong, Greer, & Brown,

1990). Children and adults with Williams syndrome exhibit abnormal responses to sounds which do not usually cause fear or discomfort to people in the general population. People with Williams syndrome may react to distressing sounds by crying, screaming, and/or covering their ears. Extreme fear responses to benign sounds, such as vacuum cleaners, motorcycles, and lawn mowers, can result in anticipatory anxiety (e.g., a child who refuses to attend school for fear of a fire drill) which disrupts daily activities. In addition, hyperacusis may be an underlying factor in the attentional deficits seen in many people with this syndrome. With age, some adults with Williams syndrome seem to become partially desensitized to distressing sounds and may be better able to tolerate noisy environments.

Williams syndrome is associated with several known medical complications and anomalies which can affect health throughout the lifespan, as shown in Table 1. Congenital cardiovascular anomalies are found in approximately 80% of people with Williams syndrome. Most often, these involve stenosis (narrowing) of blood vessels of the heart, but can include arteries going to the kidneys and other body organs. The most common cardiovascular abnormality is supravalvular aortic stenosis (SVAS) in which narrowing of the aorta disrupts blood flow. The condition often becomes more severe with age and requires careful monitoring by a cardiologist. Peripheral pulmonary artery stenosis is also common in infancy but usually improves over time.

Approximately 15% of infants with Williams syndrome have documented hypercalcemia (abnormally elevated levels of calcium in the blood). Hypercalcemia is most often transient and disappears by the fourth year of life. However, a minority of older children and adults with Williams syndrome experience persistent hypercalcemia which requires monitoring because of the potential for secondary health problems, such as calcium accumulation in the kidneys (nephrocalcinosis), related to abnormal calcium metabolism (Pober, Lacro, Rice, Mandell, & Teele, 1993).

Hypertension (high blood pressure) is present in almost half of children and adults with Williams syndrome, even in the absence of cardiovascular or renal disease (Broder et al., 1999). The etiology of hypertension in this population is unknown, and it does not appear to be related to the generalized anxiety seen in most people with the condition. Hypertension in Williams syndrome is significantly correlated with infantile hypercalcemia, potentially implicating subtle abnormalities in calcium metabolism. Abnormalities of the blood vessels due to the underlying elastin microdeletion could also theoretically contribute to hypertension in this disorder (Broder et al., 1999).

Chronic constipation is common among people with Williams syndrome and may account for stomach pain and feeding problems in infants and children. Stool softeners are often needed to maintain regularity and to avoid secondary gastrointestinal complications, such as rectal prolapse. Many older children and adults with Williams syndrome experience incontinence and urinary tract infections, sometimes related to structural bladder changes such as diverticula ("pockets" in the bladder wall) (Morris, Leonard, Dilts, & Demsey, 1990). Renal abnormalities, ranging from mild to severe, are found in approximately 18% of those affected (Pober et al., 1993).

Table 1. Medical/Developmental Characteristics of Williams Syndrome*

FINDING	AGE SEEN			INCIDENCE
	INFANT	CHILD	ADULT	
Characteristic Facial Appearance	x	x	x	
Developmental Delay	x	x		
Mental Retardation (Usually Mild)		x	x	
Cardiovascular Disease (Mostly Supravalvular Aortic Stenosis)	x	x	x	
Characteristic Cognitive Profile		x	x	
Hypotonia (Central)	x	x		Frequent: ≥75%
Loose Jointedness	x	x		
Hyperactive Deep Tendon Reflexes		x	x	
Hyperacusis	x	x	x	
Dental Abnormalities		x	x	
Soft, Stretchy Skin	x	x	x	
Prematurely Gray Hair			x	
Generalized Anxiety Disorder		x	x	
Feeding Difficulties	x	x		
Chronic Otitis Media	x	x		
Attention Deficit Hyperactivity Disorder		x		
Early Puberty		x		
Hyperopia		x	x	
Strabismus	x			
Enuresis		x		Common: 50 to <75%
Umbilical Hernia	x			
Joint Contractures	x	x	x	
Awkward Gait		x	x	
Hypertonia (Peripheral)		x	x	
Hypercalciuria	x	x	x	
Chronic Urinary Tract Infections			x	
Constipation	x	x	x	
Colon Diverticulae		x	x	Less Common: 25 to <50%
Inguinal Hernia	x			
Renal Artery Stenosis	x	x	x	
Lordosis		x	x	
Idiopathic Hypercalcemia	x		x	
Structural Urinary Tract Abnormalities	x	x	x	
Nephrocalcinosis	x	x	x	
Rectal Prolapse	x	x		
Kyphosis			x	
Hypothyroidism	x	x	x	Occasional: <25%
Diabetes Mellitus			x	
Arnold-chiari Malformation	x	x	x	
Borderline To Average Intelligence		x	x	

Although most of the associated medical issues in Williams syndrome can be successfully managed, early identification and monitoring are key for ensuring optimum health. Health care directives for people with Williams syndrome have been published and are helpful for guiding medical management of children and adults with this disorder (Committee on Genetics, 2001).

Natural History

Infants with Williams syndrome often come to medical attention because of cardiovascular abnormalities in the first year of life. Many cardiologists are familiar with the association between SVAS and Williams syndrome, and babies born with SVAS are likely to be referred for genetic testing. Individuals with other, more common types of heart defects, as well as those who are free of cardiac anomalies, are less likely to receive an early diagnosis (Huang, Sadler, O'Riordan, & Robin, 2002). Newborns with Williams syndrome tend to be relatively small in weight as compared to other babies in the family. Growth remains slow, and many infants experience failure to thrive during the first year of life. Typically, they are cranky, fussy babies in the first year, possibly related to infantile hypercalcemia and/or gastrointestinal problems.

Both motor and language development are delayed in children with Williams syndrome. Hypotonia (low muscle tone) and joint laxity are likely contributors to motor delays in young children. Older children and adults often show increased tone and stiffness. Many individuals develop contractures of both large and small joints, resulting in a crouched, awkward gait and impairments in fine motor function (Kaplan, Kirschner, Watters, & Costa, 1989). Spinal curvatures, particularly kyphosis and lordosis, are relatively common among older children and adults with Williams syndrome. Adult height is usually less than expected for the family background.

Language acquisition is delayed, and young children with Williams syndrome benefit from early intervention services, including speech therapy. As they age, however, language becomes an area of relative strength for most people with Williams syndrome. Relatively sophisticated language abilities may mask cognitive deficits in other areas, particularly visuospatial tasks. The majority of school-aged children with Williams syndrome require special education, particularly for math and reading. Most test within the mild range of mental retardation, with some individuals having average intelligence and others more severe degrees of intellectual impairment. Some adults with Williams syndrome are employed in the community, most often with the support of a job coach and/or supervision from a sponsoring agency. Many find work in traditional sheltered workshop settings. Although they may seem capable of more challenging work, a significant number of adults with Williams syndrome have difficulty maintaining competitive employment due to visuospatial deficits, distractibility, and psychiatric issues, particularly anxiety (Davies, Howlin, & Udwin, 1997; Morris, Demsey, Leonard, Dilts, & Blackburn, 1988). As with most other genetic syndromes, little is known about long-term functioning into later adulthood and old age in people with Williams syndrome. Based on the limited number of cases reported, there is no evidence for an increased incidence of Alzheimer disease, as in Down syndrome, or other neurodegenerative conditions.

Cognitive Strengths and Weaknesses

Individuals with Williams syndrome show a wide range of cognitive abilities. The average IQ among those affected is between 50 and 60, with most functioning in the mild to moderate range of intellectual disability. A small percentage of those with the syndrome test within the average range of intellectual functioning, while some fall within the severe range of mental retardation. There is significant scatter in the cognitive profile of people with Williams syndrome which cannot be fully appreciated by simply considering an overall IQ score. Relative strengths include language abilities, facial recognition, and short term auditory memory. By contrast, the syndrome is associated in most people with significant deficits in visuospatial construction, perceptual planning, and fine motor control. In practical terms, educational and vocational interventions for individuals with Williams syndrome are often complicated by their uneven abilities and associated impairments, such as hyperacusis and attentional disorders. Relatively advanced language abilities may mask cognitive impairments and give the impression of higher overall functioning. Visuospatial deficits coupled with fine motor difficulties may make it impossible for a person to Williams syndrome to perform a work task which he or she can otherwise describe in exacting detail. Research is currently focused on identifying and describing specific aspects of the Williams syndrome cognitive profile. Such efforts will ideally lead to the development of appropriate strategies and interventions to address their educational needs in the future.

Language

Williams syndrome has been a source of great interest to researchers studying the connection between intelligence and language. Some studies of Williams syndrome show preserved language abilities in the context of significantly impaired cognition, calling into question the interdependency of the two (Bellugi, Wang, & Jernigan, 1994). Vocabulary, for example, appears to be a relative strength for individuals with Williams syndrome, although discrepancies between verbal and nonverbal abilities may not become apparent until later childhood or adolescence (Jarrold, Baddeley, & Hewes, 1998). In most people with Williams syndrome, however, vocabulary still falls below that of CA-(chronological age) matched controls without mental retardation. Some studies have shown grammar (the ordering of words in a sentence) and other aspects of syntax to be areas of strength for people with Williams syndrome (Bellugi et al., 1994), while other researchers have confirmed significant impairments in syntax as compared with CA-matched, and in some cases, MA (mental age)-matched controls (Karmiloff-Smith et al., 1997; Volterra, Capirci, Pezzini, Sabbadini, & Vicari, 1996).

Studies have also shown conflicting results with regard to semantics, that is, the meaning and organization of words. Anecdotally, people with Williams syndrome prefer the use of unusual words and phrases in conversation. Unusual word choices were confirmed by Bellugi, Wang, and Jernigan (1994) who found that adolescents and adults with Williams syndrome produced more low-frequency words than MA-matched controls on word fluency tests. When asked to name as many animals as possible in a 60 second period, for example, children with Williams syndrome included uncommon animals such as ibex, condor, and saber-toothed tiger among their choices. Subsequent studies by other research groups (Scott et al., 1995; Volterra et al., 1996) found no differences between children with Williams syndrome and MA-matched controls on word fluency tasks, suggesting that semantic abilities in people with this disorder are commensurate with cognitive functioning.

The debate over language in Williams syndrome continues and may be resolved by further research. Most researchers agree that while linguistic abilities may not be completely spared, certain aspects of language represent areas of relative strength for people with Williams syndrome, at least as compared to those with similar levels of cognitive impairment. In addition, exaggerated linguistic affect may give a false impression of highly developed language abilities in people with Williams syndrome. Their use of exclamations, dramatic inflection, and other storytelling devices creates interest and adds to their positive interactive style.

Musical Ability

Only a handful of studies have formally examined the musical abilities of individuals with Williams syndrome. Comparable levels of musical interest were found among children with Down syndrome and those with Williams syndrome, although those in the latter group were more likely to play an instrument (Hodapp, Dykens, Fidler, & Rosner, 2000). Rhythmic abilities among some children with Williams syndrome were found to be equal to those of typically developing controls (Levitan & Bellugi, 1998), with the Williams group showing an impressive ability to improvise. Musical abilities among people with this syndrome may in part be related to hypertimbria, an enhanced ability to distinguish the subjective quality of a sound (e.g., different musical instruments playing the same note). Anecdotally, parents report that their children with Williams syndrome have an uncanny ability to identify the exact origin of sounds in their environment (e.g., distinguishing different types of aircraft based on their engine sounds). This may be a variant of perfect pitch, the ability to precisely recognize musical notes, which in turn could be related to the known association between Williams syndrome and hyperacusis. Although these preliminary studies and observations are intriguing, further research is needed to determine the extent to which musical abilities are part of the Williams syndrome phenotype.

Visuospatial Perception

Visuospatial perception refers to the ability to process and interpret visual information related to the location of objects in space. Deficits in this cognitive function have a practical impact a wide range of daily activities, from drawing and writing to tying shoelaces. People with Williams syndrome tend to perform very poorly on visuospatial tasks as compared to both typically developing children and those with other types of developmental disabilities, such as Down syndrome (Mervis, Morris, Bertrand, & Robinson, 1999). Impairments in motor planning, spatial orientation, and eye-hand coordination may explain their difficulty with relatively simple tasks, such as orienting blocks to match a model (Dykens, Hodapp, & Finucane, 2000). Several studies have shown that children with Williams syndrome have severe perceptual-motor deficits on tests which require figure copying and drawing. Bellugi, Wang, and Jernigan (1994) asked children with Williams syndrome to both describe and draw specific objects and animals. Their verbal descriptions were richly detailed and accurate, but their drawings were disorganized and unrecognizable.

Debate continues as to whether this represents an age-related delay in drawing development or a syndrome-specific area of abnormal cognitive functioning. Recent studies have suggested that visuospatial deficits in Williams syndrome may be localized to the parieto-occipital region of the brain which is believed to process visual information related to space and motion. By contrast, preliminary research suggests that people with Williams syndrome are adequately able to process visual information about the form and color of objects, a skill believed to be mediated by the temporal region of the brain. For example, Nakamura, Kaneoke, Watanabe, and Kakigi (2002) found that performance on line copying tasks improved in a small cohort of children with Williams syndrome when colored dots were used as guides. Such research suggests that efforts to better understand the underlying pathophysiology of cognitive deficits in Williams syndrome may eventually lead to practical interventions.

Behavior and Personality

People with Williams syndrome have long been noted to be friendly and outgoing. These positive personality attributes are mentioned in even the earliest reports of the syndrome and have become a hallmark of the behavioral phenotype. Some researchers have speculated that the friendly demeanor in Williams syndrome can be partly explained by its characteristic facial appearance, which includes a wide mouth, upturned nose, and a stellate iris pattern resulting in "sparkly," animated eyes. People with Williams syndrome tend to have an unusual interest in faces from an early age, and research has confirmed a relative strength in their ability to recognize and remember faces (Bellugi, Wang, and Jernigan, 1994). This interest, combined with their heightened linguistic affect, gives the impression of an attentive, charming, and enthusiastic listener (Levine & Wharton, 2001). Families report that their children with Williams syndrome are often the "greeters" at social functions, initiating conversation and asking social questions ("What's your name? Where are you from?") to newcomers. Their attractive, happy appearance may also engender positive, friendly reactions from those who interact with them, reinforcing outgoing, gregarious behavior from an early age. Williams syndrome is therefore an excellent model for how inherent physical and personality characteristics can become reinforced and even exaggerated through the environmental responses they generate.

Individuals with Williams syndrome come across as unusually empathic and emotionally sensitive. Researchers have speculated that they may have an intact "theory of mind," that is, the ability to take on the perspective and infer the mental state of another person. This ability is known to be impaired in people with autism and other types of developmental disabilities. People with Williams syndrome have been found to perform better than MA-matched controls, and in some cases as well as typical peers, on various tasks designed to assess theory of mind (Karmiloff-Smith, Klima, Bellugi, Grant, & Baron-Cohen, 1995; Tager-Flusberg, Boshart, & Baron-Cohen, 1998). These findings support the anecdotal impression of a sensitive, caring personality phenotype in Williams syndrome.

Despite charming and friendly personalities, many people with Williams syndrome have difficulty with social interaction. They are sometimes overly friendly, even with strangers, to the point that their social style becomes intrusive. They may be socially uninhibited, leading to indiscriminate and inappropriate interactions with others. They frequently have difficulty sustaining friendships, in part because they "come on too strong" and tend to become infatuated with friends. They can also be emotionally labile and physically over-demonstrative, putting them at risk for sexual exploitation. Children and adults with Williams syndrome can benefit from social skills training (e.g., role playing, structured interactions) to help them understand social boundaries (Davies, Udwin, & Howlin, 1998).

Associated Psychopathology

Over the course of their lifetimes, most individuals with Williams syndrome meet the criteria for both mental retardation and at least one psychiatric disorder. Some of the associated psychopathology seems to be age-related. Young children with Williams syndrome are often diagnosed with Attention Deficit Hyperactivity Disorder, while motor hyperactivity rarely persists into adulthood. Adults continue to have short attention spans and distractibility, however, even in the absence of hyperactivity.

Anxiety disorders are common among both children and adults with Williams syndrome. Over half of those studied using standard psychiatric interviews were considered chronic "worriers," while almost all had some persistent anxiety-producing fears (Dykens, 2000). Specific phobias are often related to noise (e.g., thunder, motorcycles), natural disasters, illness, and fears about the future. The high incidence of phobias in Williams syndrome contrasts strongly with the relatively low prevalence (<5%) of these conditions in people with nonspecific mental retardation. By contrast, autistic symptoms are only rarely seen in association with Williams syndrome. Many of the characteristic behavioral features of autism and Williams syndrome are mutually exclusive (e.g., poor versus intact theory of mind, facial emotion recognition, language). Some autism researchers have a keen interest in studying Williams syndrome because its many contrasting characteristics could potentially provide insights into the underlying neurological basis for autism.

As with most other genetic syndromes, there have been virtually no controlled trials to study the effectiveness of specific medications on psychiatric symptoms in Williams syndrome. Pharmacological treatment is symptomatic and may include stimulant drugs for attentional disorders as well as anti-anxiety medications. Non-pharmacological strategies include reassurance, counseling, and cognitive-behavioral approaches which capitalize on the linguistic and musical strengths of people with the syndrome (Dykens, Hodapp, and Finucane, 2000). Because of the complexity of their medical, sensory, behavioral, and intellectual needs, children and adults with Williams syndrome usually require a long-term coordinated network of multidisciplinary supports. Fortunately, the many positive aspects of the behavioral phenotype foster a high degree of dedication and interest among caregivers who often consider it a privilege to work with these unique and fascinating individuals.

Resources

Williams Syndrome Association
PO Box 297, Clawson, MI 48017-0297
Phone: 248-541-3630
800-806-1871 (toll-free)
Fax: 248-541-3631
Website: www.williams-syndrome.org
Email: info@williams-syndrome.org

The Lili Claire Foundation
2800 28th Street, Suite 325, Santa Monica, CA 90405
Phone: 310-396-4355
Fax: 310-396-2127
Website: www.liliclairefoundation.org
Email: staff@liliclairefoundation.org

Publications

Williams Syndrome: Approaches to Intervention
by Eleanor Semel and Sue R. Rosner
Published by Lawrence Erlbaum Associates, Mahwah, NJ
January 2003

Journey from Cognition to Brain to Gene: Perspectives from Williams Syndrome
by Ursula Bellugi (ed.) and Marie St. George
Published by MIT Press, Cambridge, MA
November 2001

References

Bellugi, U., Wang, P., & Jernigan, T. L. (1994). Williams syndrome: An unusual neuropsychological profile. In S. H. Browman and J. Grafram (Eds.), *Atypical cognitive deficits in developmental disorders* (pp. 23-56). Mahwah, NJ: Lawrence Erlbaum Associates.

Beuren, A. J., Apitz, J., & Harmjanz, D. (1962). Supravalvular aortic stenosis in association with mental retardation and a certain facial appearance. *Circulation, 26,* 1235-1240.

Broder, K., Reinhardt, E., Ahern, J., Lifton, R., Tamborlane, W., & Pober, B. (1999). Elevated ambulatory blood pressure in 20 subjects with Williams syndrome. *American Journal of Medical Genetics, 83,* 356-360.

Committee on Genetics, American Academy of Pediatrics. (2001). Health care supervision for children with Williams syndrome. *Pediatrics, 107,* 1192-1204.

Davies, M., Howlin, P., & Udwin, O. (1997). Independence and adaptive behavior in adults with Williams syndrome. *American Journal of Medical Genetics, 70,* 188-195.

Davies, M., Udwin, O., & Howlin, P. (1998). Adults with Williams syndrome. *British Journal of Psychiatry, 172,* 273-276.

Dykens, E. M. (2000). *Anxiety, fears, and phobias in Williams syndrome.* Manuscript submitted for publication.

Dykens, E. M., Hodapp, R. M., & Finucane, B. M. (2000). Williams syndrome. In *Genetics and mental retardation syndromes: A new look at behavior and interventions* (pp.97-135). Baltimore, MD: Paul H. Brookes Publishing Company.

Ewart, A. K., Morris, C. A., Atkinson, D., Jin, W., Sternes, K., Spallone, P., et al. (1993). Hemizygosity at the elastin locus in a developmental disorder, Williams syndrome. *Nature Genetics, 5,* 11-16.

Frangiskakis, J. M., Ewart, A. K., Morris, C. A., Mervis, C. B., Bertrand, J., Robinson, B. F., et al. (1996). LIM-kinase1 hemizygosity implicated in impaired visuospatial constructive cognition. *Cell, 86,* 59-69.

Hodapp, R. M., Dykens, E. M., Fidler, D. J., & Rosner, B. A. (2000). *Social competence in children with Williams versus Down syndromes.* Submitted for publication.

Huang, L., Sadler, L., O'Riordan, M. A., & Robin, N. H. (2002). Delay in diagnosis of Williams syndrome. *Clinical Pediatrics, 41,* 257-261.

Jarrold, C., Baddeley, A. D., & Hewes, A. K. (1998). Verbal and nonverbal abilities in the Williams syndrome phenotype: Evidence for diverging developmental trajectories. *Journal of Child Psychology and Psychiatry and Allied Disciplines, 39,* 511-523.

Kaplan, P., Kirschner, M., Watters, G., & Costa, M. T. (1989). Contractures in patients with Williams syndrome. *Pediatrics, 84,* 895-899.

Kapp, M. E., von Noorden, G. K., & Jenkins, R. (1995). Strabismus in Williams syndrome. *American Journal of Ophthalmology, 119,* 355-360.

Karmiloff-Smith, A., Grant, J., Berthoud, I., Davies, M., Howlin, P., & Udwin, O. (1997). Language and Williams syndrome: How intact is "intact"? *Child Development, 68,* 246-262.

Karmiloff-Smith, A., Klima, E., Bellugi, U., Grant, J., & Baron-Cohen, S. (1995). Is there a social processing module? Language, face processing, and theory of mind in individuals with Williams syndrome. *Journal of Cognitive Neuroscience, 7,* 196-208.

Klein, A. J., Armstrong, B. L., Greer, M. K., & Brown, F. R. 3rd. (1990). Hyperacusis and otitis media in individuals with Williams syndrome. *Journal of Speech and Hearing Disorders, 55,* 339-344.

Levine, K., & Wharton, R. (2001). Williams syndrome and happiness. *American Journal on Mental Retardation, 105,* 363-371.

Levitan, D. J., & Bellugi, U. (1998). Musical abilities in individuals with Williams syndrome. *Music Perception, 15,* 357-398.

Mervis, C. B., Morris, C. A., Bertrand, J., & Robinson, B. F. (1999). Williams syndrome: Findings from an integrated program of research. In H. Tager-Flusberg (Ed.), *Neurodevelopmental disorders: Contributions to a framework from the cognitive sciences* (pp. 65-110). Cambridge, MA: MIT Press.

Morris, C. A., Demsey, S. A., Leonard, C. O., Dilts, C., & Blackburn, B. L. (1988). Natural history of Williams syndrome: Physical characteristics. *Journal of Pediatrics, 113,* 318-326.

Morris, C. A., Leonard, C. O., Dilts, C., & Demsey, S. A. (1990). Adults with Williams syndrome. *American Journal of Medical Genetics, 6 (Suppl),* 102-107.

Morris, C. A., Thomas, I. T., & Greenberg, F. (1993). Williams syndrome: Autosomal dominant inheritance. *American Journal of Medical Genetics, 47,* 478-481.

Nakamura, M., Kaneoke, Y., Watanabe, K., & Kakigi, R. (2002). Visual information process in Williams syndrome: Intact motion detection accompanied by typical visuospatial dysfunctions. *European Journal of Neuroscience, 16,* 1810-1818.

Pober, B. R., Lacro, R. V., Rice, C., Mandell, V., & Teele, R. L. (1993). Renal findings in 40 individuals with Williams syndrome. *American Journal of Medical Genetics, 46,* 271-274.

Preus, M. (1984). The Williams syndrome: Objective definition and diagnosis. *Clinical Genetics, 25,* 422-428.

Scott, P., Mervis, C. B., Bertrand, J., Klein, B. P., Armstrong, S. C., & Ford, A. J. (1995). Semantic organization and word fluency in 9- and 10-year-old children with Williams syndrome. *Genetic Counseling, 6,* 172-173.

Stromme, P., Bjornstad, P. G., & Ramstad, K. (2002). Prevalence estimation of Williams syndrome. *Journal of Child Neurology, 17,* 269-271.

Tager-Flusberg, H., Boshart, J., & Baron-Cohen, S. (1998). Reading the windows to the soul: Evidence of domain-specific sparing in Williams syndrome. *Journal of Cognitive Neuroscience, 10,* 631-639.

Volterra, V., Capirci, O., Pezzini, G., Sabbadini, L., & Vicari, S. (1996). Linguistic abilities in Italian children with Williams syndrome. *Cortex, 32,* 663-677.

Williams, J. C., Barrett-Boyes, B. G., & Lowe, J. B. (1961). Supravalvular aortic stenosis. *Circulation, 24,* 1311-1318.

Wu, Y. Q., Sutton, V. R., Nickerson, E., Lupski, J. R., Potocki, L., Korenberg, J. R., et al. (1998). Delineation of the common critical region in Williams syndrome and clinical correlation of growth, heart defects, ethnicity, and parental origin. *American Journal of Medical Genetics, 78,* 82-89.

CHAPTER 5

Smith-Magenis Syndrome

Elliott W. Simon

Introduction

A characteristic behavioral phenotype that results from the interplay among bio-medical, psychological and psychosocial factors is perhaps more evident in Smith-Magenis syndrome (SMS) than in any other genetically based mental retardation syndrome. Our growing understanding of these factors and their interrelationship is beginning to drive treatment for SMS and other genetically based developmental disorders from a new syndromic-based approach (Simon & Finucane, 1998). SMS is a newly identified genetic disorder (Smith et al., 1986) with a characteristic pattern of facial features, sensory deficits, sleep disorder, neurological findings, mental retardation, and behavioral presentation that includes self-injury. Through the study of affected individuals we have already gained a better understanding of how biomedical factors can impact psychological, cognitive, behavioral, and psychosocial functioning.

Etiology/Incidence

SMS is a chromosome deletion syndrome, a portion of one of the two number 17 chromosomes is missing or deleted. Individuals with SMS therefore have one normal and one affected chromosome 17 in each of their cells. SMS is also termed a continuous gene syndrome. This means that the missing genetic material is continuous on the chromosome, and in the case of SMS, varying numbers of genes in this region may be missing. Although the missing genes in SMS are positioned close to each other they may have very different functions. This results in a complex physical and behavioral phenotype. The missing genes in SMS are in the region known as 17p11.2 and are only detectable by high resolution chromosome analysis. Because of this, karyotype analyses, which confirm gross genetic findings such as the extra chromosome 21 in Down syndrome, will not reveal the SMS deletion. This, along with a lack of knowledge of the syndrome has resulted in an under-diagnosis of affected individuals.

Almost all cases of SMS are the result of deletions that are not inherited and the chance of a parent having a second child with SMS is usually no greater than for an individual who has not had a child with SMS. There have been a few cases of essentially asymptomatic individuals who are mosaic for the deletion (the deletion is not present in all cells) bearing children with the full SMS (Zori et al., 1993). Because of this, parents of SMS individuals should have a complete molecular genetic work-up.

The general incidence statistic for SMS is 1/25,000 live births (Greenberg et al., 1991). SMS is, however, under-diagnosed (Lockwood et al., 1988) and the incidence of SMS may be very common in individuals with mental retardation. During a five year period in a population of approximately 1,000 individuals with mental retardation 23 people were diagnosed with SMS (Finucane & Simon, 1999).

Physical and Medical Findings

SMS has a constellation of typical physical characteristics and medical findings. These include facial and body morphologies as well as specific neurological findings. While some of these physical and medical features are benign others are related to the behavioral characteristics of SMS.

Infants with SMS have significant low muscle tone and are characterized as floppy babies. Poor eating during infancy may result in some SMS babies being diagnosed with failure to thrive. Other cranio-facial findings include under-developed cheekbones, a low nasal bridge, unusually formed ears, abnormalities of the palate (at times cleft), a prominent jaw in older children and adults, a down turned mouth and a protruding upper lip (Lockwood et al., 1988; Smith et al., 1986). Skeletal characteristics include short fingers and toes, broad hands, webbing of the toes (particularly toes 2 and 3), fingertip pads, abnormal palmar creases, scoliosis, and a small stature. See Figure 1.

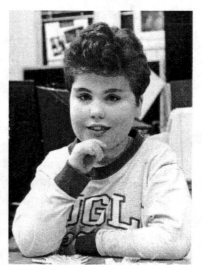

Figure 1.

Neurologically, abnormal EEG patterns and seizures have been reported, though are not considered a hallmark of SMS. Brain malformations can be present in individuals with SMS though none have been reported with any significant frequency. In the Greenberg et al. (1996) study, 52% of SMS individuals were found to have some brain malformation including a partial absence of vermis and dystrophic calcifications of the frontal lobe. An important neurological finding with behavioral implications for the self-injury present in SMS is a decreased sensitivity to pain and reduced deep tendon reflexes with peripheral neuropathy (Greenberg et al., 1991; Greenberg et al., 1996, Zori et al., 1993). Peripheral neuropathies are characterized by reduced and abnormal sensations in the extremities.

Visual system findings include strabismus and nearsightedness (Finucane, Jaeger, Kurtz, Weinstein, & Scott, 1993; Chen, Lupski, Greenberg, & Lewis, 1996). The Finucane et al. (1993) study reported 10 individuals with retinal detachment. The precise interplay of the eye abnormalities and self-injury, which may result in retinal detachment, is as yet unclear. However, individuals with SMS should be considered at risk for retinal detachment especially as they enter adolescence. Hearing deficits and recurrent otitis media are also common if not almost universal in SMS (Greenberg et al., 1996). The relationship among otitis media, self-injury, and hearing loss is beginning to be elucidated. The facial and palate structure of individuals with SMS results in a reduction in sinus cavity capacity. This increases the susceptibility to otitis media that may in turn play a part in the genesis of self injurious head banging. This combination may in many cases cause severe hearing loss.

Cardiac and renal findings are also prevalent in SMS. Greenberg et al. (1996) found kidney abnormalities (including ectopic kidneys and renal agenesis) in 35% of people studied and cardiac malformations (including mitral regurgitation septal defects and aortic stenosis) in 37%. If a diagnosis of SMS is not made, these medical conditions may go undiagnosed with resulting permanent damage. This is especially true for the renal findings.

Based upon these physical and medical findings, an accepted medical protocol has been developed for the initial and annual physical examination of individuals with SMS (GeneClinics, 2002) See Table 1.

Table 1. Recommended physical exam for SMS (GeneClinics, 2002)

Newly Diagnosed
- Physical and neurological exam
- Renal ultrasound
- Audiological evaluation
- Spinal radiographs
- Opthomological evaluation
- Otolaryngological evaluation
- Echocardiogram
- Assessment for velopharyngeal incompetence
- Routine blood chemistries
- Quantitative Immunoglobulins
- Fasting lipid profile
- Thyroid function

Annual Evaluations
- Routine physical
- Thyroid function
- Fasting lipid profile
- Urinalysis
- Scoliosis
- Opthomology
- Audiological

Behavioral and Psychological Phenotype

The cognitive and behavioral aspects of SMS have been called the most salient characteristics of the syndrome (Smith, Dykens, & Greenberg, 1998a). These features include a specific pattern of self-injury, stereotypies, and developmental delay. A severe sleep disorder is also present in many individuals with SMS and complicates behavioral and psychiatric presentations.

Self-Injury

A wide array of specific self injurious behaviors have been reported in individuals with SMS. These include hand and wrist biting, head banging, skin picking, hair pulling, and slapping self (Colley, Leversha, Voullaire, & Rogers, 1990; Dykens & Smith, 1998; Greenberg et al., 1991 & 1996; Smith, Dykens, & Greenberg, 1998a). In addition, these researchers have reported two characteristic self-injuries, picking at fingernails and toenails until they bleed (onychotillomania) and inserting objects in body orifices (polyembolokoilomania). The severity of self-injury can become quite intense. In some cases, toenails and fingernails have been completely removed, retinal detachment has occurred and object insertion has necessitated surgical removal of the object from the nose or ear or has led to serious infection.

Two recent studies (Dykens & Smith, 1998; Finucane, Dirrigl, & Simon; 2001) have found the prevalence of self-injury in SMS to be over 90%, with hand and wrist biting the most common single behavior. Onychotillomania and polyembolokoilomania have been reported in between a third to a half of individuals.

The developmental course of self-injury in SMS has also recently begun to be described. Greenberg et al. (1991) described onychotillomania as uncommon under the age of 5 or 6 years. Finucane, Dirrigl, and Simon (2001) found that about 25% of parents of SMS children under the age of 12 reported onychotillomania while 85% of the parents of older SMS children reported this behavior. Age-related increases in slapping self and skin picking were also noted.

Stereotypies

Dykens, Finucane, and Gayley (1997) utilized the *Reiss Screen of Maladaptive Behavior* (Reiss, 1988) and determined that 7 of the 10 individuals with SMS in their sample engaged in unusual motor movements. Most common were the "self-hug" and "lick and flip." The self-hug was first described by Finucane et al. (1994) and is usually exhibited when an individual with SMS is happy or excited. The behavior has been observed more frequently in children than adults and is described as a midline tic-like movement. Some individuals wrap their arms around their chests as if hugging themselves and then tense their bodies in quick tic-like movements. Other individuals clasp their hands together in front of their bodies in a twisting motion quickly pressing both clasped hands against their chest tensing their body while grimacing facially. The movements appear involuntary and often occur in quick spasmodic like flurries. Although this behavior does not interfere with purposeful hand use it is an important diagnostic marker and should prompt an evaluation for SMS.

Dykens, Finucane, and Gayley (1997) also reported an unusual repetitive behavior they termed the "lick and flip." Nine of ten individuals engaged in a repetitive sequence of page turning when testing materials were placed in front of them. This sequence involved an exaggerated wetting of the fingers by placing four fingers of one hand in their mouth and then using the wetted hand to turn pages in succession.

Other Maladaptive Behavior

Aside from the characteristic self-injury profile, individuals with SMS engage in many additional behaviors that interfere with their adaptive functioning. Hyperactivity, tantrums, attention seeking, aggressive and destructive behaviors have been reported as present in as high as 80% of individuals with SMS (Dykens, Finucane, & Gayley, 1997; Greenberg et al., 1996, Smith et al., 1986).

Sleep Disturbance

Another hallmark of the SMS is an almost universal sleep disturbance (Smith, Dykens, & Greenberg; 1998a). The presence of this sleep disturbance may do much to exacerbate the behavioral profile. Control of the sleep disturbance, though very difficult, can aid in supporting the individual with SMS and impact positively on their quality of life.

The sleep disturbance in SMS is pervasive and expressed in several sleep domains. Dykens and Smith (1998) determined that the presence of a sleep disorder was the strongest predictor of problem behaviors. Most individuals with SMS have difficulty falling asleep, are easily wakened and once awake find it difficult to fall back asleep. Individuals with SMS also take frequent naps during the day. Although the biology of the SMS sleep disorder remains unknown, researchers have postulated a melatonin deficit hypothesis. Melatonin is a hormone that is involved in the regulation of an individual's circadian rhythm.

De Leersnyder and Munnich (1999) studied 20 children with SMS between the ages of 4 and 17. She found that all of the children were asleep by 9 p.m., had frequent awakenings and were awake before dawn. Children had frequent daytime naps and all were very tired by dinnertime. De Leersnyder and Munnich (1999) monitored 24-hour melatonin levels in 8 of the children. In the normal course of melatonin, levels of the hormone rise from 9 p.m., peak at midnight and taper off until dawn. The 8 children with SMS evidenced a reverse pattern, melatonin levels rose during the morning hours and peaked at noon. De Leersnyder and Munnich (1999) believe that the hyperactivity with which some individuals with SMS present is due to fighting against sleep.

Treating the sleep disorder in SMS with oral administration of melatonin has had mixed results according to anecdotal reports. Hagerman (1999a) suggests that people with SMS evidencing a sleep disturbance should receive a melatonin trial of 3 mg at bedtime. She further states that if melatonin is ineffective then a trial of clonidine or trazodone at bedtime should be considered. Alternatively, it has also been suggested that as the light sensitive pineal gland is involved in melatonin regulation, that light therapy would be of benefit. Smith, Dykens, and Greenberg (1998b) report on one such successful treatment in a 6 year old who responded to 20 minutes of light therapy administered each morning at 6 a.m. beginning in January. Dramatic improvement was noted in behavioral and sleep problems. In May of the same year, the light therapy was decreased to 10 minutes per day with an increase in behavioral problems. When light therapy was increased to 15 minutes per day behavior improved within 48 hours.

Cognition

Cognitive developmental delay in individuals with SMS is evident very early in life. Most individuals with SMS are assessed to function within the mild and moderate levels of mental retardation, although there can be large variability in IQ score and adaptive levels.

In one of the few examinations of the cognitive profiles of individuals with SMS, Dykens, Finucane, and Gayley (1997) administered a series of cognitive and intellectual measures to 10 individuals with SMS. All 10 individuals evidenced a weakness in sequential processing skills. Sequential processing involves the ability to place items in an order and to remember lists of auditory and visual stimuli. Deficits in these abilities may be related to underlying processing problems or to the hyperactivity and inattention observed in individuals with SMS. Simultaneous processing skills, such as naming a partially completed drawing, were a relative strength for these individuals. Simultaneous processing involves the ability to perceive a whole from its parts. Strengths were also found in long-term memory for places, people and things and letter/word recognition. Expressive language development was higher than would be predicted based on their overall level of cognitive functioning.

Social

The social characteristics of individuals with SMS have been the focus of few controlled investigations. Social adaptive skills as measured by standardized assessments are delayed, with researchers (Dykens, Finucane, & Gayley, 1997; Greenberg et al., 1996) finding an average socialization age of approximately 5 years. People with SMS are very demanding attention seekers and have difficulty in sustaining attention. This aspect of their behavior impinges negatively on their social interactions. In addition, children with SMS seek adult as opposed to peer attention and are very sensitive to the emotional state of others. The social behavioral phenotype of SMS is based largely on anecdotal reports from teachers and caregivers. Many of these reports have appeared in the SPECTRUM newsletter, the official newsletter of the national support group for SMS, Parents and Researchers Interested in Smith Magenis Syndrome (PRISMS) and in GENETWORK, the newsletter of the Genetics Department at Elwyn Inc., Elwyn, PA.

Haas-Givler and her colleagues (1994; 1995; 1996) have reported on observations of the social behavior of children with SMS from the perspective of a classroom special education teacher. Haas-Givler characterizes the SMS child as an insatiable attention seeker who is adult oriented, extremely affectionate and who is very sensitive to the emotions of others. She reports that this affection is sometimes inappropriately overly demonstrative, with indiscriminate hugging of strangers and known adults in a bone crushing grip. She notes that this need for attention is often times at the root of behavioral disturbances in the classroom. This is due to diminishing attention at some point with the result often being self-injury or tantrums escalating to aggression. Other characteristics that she has observed in the classroom include responsiveness to routine and structure, an eagerness to please and communicate through sign, communication board or speech and a developed sense of humor. SMS children are easily motivated by food, sticker rewards and attention. She also reports observations of a fascination with electronics, calculators and computers.

Psychiatric Disorders

Given the behavioral presentation of individuals with SMS it is no surprise that many meet the DSM-IV (American Psychiatric Association, 1994) criteria for and are diagnosed with psychiatric disorders. Dykens, Finucane, and Gayley (1997) found 6 of 10 SMS individuals with clinically significant psychopathology scores on the Reiss Screen (Reiss, 1988). There has been no systematic examination of the prevalence of psychiatric disorders in a large cohort of individuals with SMS, however, case reports and behavioral studies do mention the presence of multiple psychiatric disorders: Attention Deficit Hyperactivity Disorder, Pervasive Developmental Disorder NOS, and Cyclical Mood Disorders.

Difficulties with attention and hyperactivity result in many children with SMS being diagnosed with attention deficit disorder and or hyperactivity disorder. The high prevalence of self-injury and stereotypies coupled with a failure to develop peer relationships appropriate to their developmental level, language delay and overall general developmental delay also results in many children meeting the criteria for Pervasive Developmental Disorder NOS. The sociability and attention craving of individuals with SMS usually obviates a diagnosis of autistic disorder, although Vostanis, Harrington, Prendergast and Farndon (1994) do report on a 14 year old boy with SMS who met the DSM-III-R (American Psychiatric Association, 1987) criteria for autistic disorder.

Individuals with SMS have also been characterized as having difficulty in regulating affect. Dykens and Smith (1998) found that individuals with SMS are particularly emotionally labile when compared to individuals with intellectual disability of mixed etiology and to individuals with Prader-Willi syndrome. Anecdotal reports of quickly changing affect with tantrum and aggression followed by over-apologetic behavior coupled with the high prevalence of sleep disturbance has also resulted in individuals being diagnosed with cyclical mood disorders.

Support Approaches

There are no substitutes for good psychiatry, behavioral and family support, and medical management in the treatment of individuals with SMS. Knowing that an individual has SMS makes good practice in these areas easier and a detailing of the behavioral and psychiatric phenotype of SMS is occurring quickly. Given the short time that SMS has been a recognized disorder, and consequently the short time that a phenotype has been able to be determined, there is already a rich literature for the clinician to draw on in developing a system of supports.

In my clinical experience as a psychologist, once a diagnosis is suspected through behavioral and physical observations I work closely with a team of professionals to develop a support plan for the individual. In addition to the team members that are indicated by the behavioral, cognitive, educational, vocational and physical needs of the individual it is most helpful to include as a team consultant a genetic counselor who specializes in genetic mental retardation disorders. The inclusion of this professional serves to educate members of the individual's habilitative team who may not be familiar with SMS, discuss the known features with the individual, their family and other interested parties as well as promote a linkage with the national support group PRISMS. As the habilitation team becomes familiar with SMS and is guided to utilize the available knowledge base and ongoing support provided by the SMS community, it becomes focused in its approach and the difficult treatment planning process of developing a unified integrated interdisciplinary biopsychosocial approach. Oftentimes in support planning for individuals with developmental delay and behavioral/psychiatric disorders, families, psychiatrists, primary physicians, behavior analysts, social workers, educators and vocational counselors work in isolation and opposition. Refocusing the team approach around supporting an individual with SMS helps to bring all individuals a knowledge base and approach that is more specific than the often used generic approaches to supporting individuals with dual diagnoses.

Much progress has been made in detailing the phenotype of SMS. However, little research has been completed that investigates specific interventions targeted for the SMS behavioral phenotype. Much of the specific SMS intervention knowledge is still anecdotal. It is crucial that the efficacy of specific behavioral, psychopharmacological and educational interventions be assessed for SMS individuals. Such research would enable the development of specific interventions and intervention hierarchies targeted for the SMS behavioral phenotype. Although we still may be a long way from specific SMS clinical pathways there are certain intervention approaches that logically follow from a thorough knowledge of the SMS.

Educational

Educational and teaching strategies should build on the strengths and meet the needs of an individual. The Kaufman Assessment Battery for children (Kaufman & Kaufman, 1984) or Kaufman Intelligence Test for Adolescents and Adults (Kaufman & Kaufman, 1992) should be part of a comprehensive educational assessment for individuals with SMS. As Dykens, Finucane, and Gayley (1997) have shown a specific SMS cognitive processing style, it is important to know the extent to which a given individual fits the syndromic profile of strength in long term memory and weakness in sequential processing abilities. Once a comprehensive educational assessment is completed it should form the basis for an Individualized Education Plan (IEP).

Based on the observations of Haas-Givler and Finucane (1996), several strategies can be used to promote an IEP that best utilizes the syndromic strengths of SMS. Table 2 presents the basics of this approach. A calm consistent classroom is crucial to providing an environment that promotes learning. As children with SMS are very sensitive to the emotional state of others, exaggerated emotional expressions by the teacher can serve to trigger a behavioral outburst or distract the attention of the SMS child from the lesson. Exaggerated positive or negative teacher emotions can be problematical. The teacher who constantly praises even the most minute accomplishment in an effervescent way can serve to over-excite the SMS child. Likewise, exaggerated negative emotional expression can serve to trigger tantrum or self-injury. Instructions are best given in a neutral tone without over exaggeration. SMS children should certainly be praised for accomplishments but it should be done in a way that does not result in over stimulation. A neutral tone calling attention to the accomplishment and task at hand is best. Likewise when correction is being used, minimal attention to the error and emphasis on the correct answer is preferred. The attention seeking behavior of SMS children is best controlled in classes with a small pupil size as classmates are viewed as competitors for the teacher's attention. Class sizes of between 5 to 7 pupils are suggested with one teacher and one teacher's aide.

Table 2. Recommended classroom strategies for children with SMS. (Haas-Givler & Finucane, 1996).

Classroom Strategies

- ◆ Calm Consistent Classroom
- ◆ Small Class Size
- ◆ Visual Reminders
- ◆ Reinforcers and Motivators
- ◆ Behavioral Interventions

The sequential processing deficit results in difficulty with following multi-step instructions and weaknesses in mathematical abilities. Multi-step verbal task instructions or directions are difficult for SMS children to process and execute. A series of instructions such as "pick up the paper, throw it in the trash and return to your seat" can be impossible for SMS children to completely process. Instructions are best given in simple single step phrases. The use of pictures and any visual aids possible to represent the steps of a task can greatly aid instruction. Picture schedules for activities are also useful, as a child finishes one aspect of a task, the next aspect can be pointed to on the task schedule. This also allows the teacher to better control the child's needs for attention and assure that each task of a sequence is completed correctly. The use of computers and educational software should be considered, as SMS children are intrigued with this modality. Special adaptations and simplifications of the keyboard and assuring that the monitor is of a high enough quality and large enough size to accommodate any visual problems must be taken into consideration.

The use of reinforcers to promote learning in the classroom is a necessity with most SMS children and many of them will also need a formalized classroom behavioral support plan to address problem behaviors. Attention, as one would expect, is highly valued by SMS individuals and can be implicated in some way in many behavioral outbursts. Judicious use of one-on one attention is an important classroom management technique for SMS children. The teacher must be aware that paying "one-to-one attention" to another classmate without the SMS child having a preferable activity to do may result in problem behavior. SMS children are at their best, behaviorally, when involved in a preferable one-to-one activity with an adult. Teachers must also be aware that when the one-to-one activity ends, the probability of a behavioral outburst is high, especially if the withdrawal of attention is sudden. Slow withdrawal of the one-to-one attention and substitution of the attention with a pre-ferred solo activity is a strategy to avoid the attention withdrawal motivated tantrum.

For learning motivation and reinforcement, visual rewards and attention are pre-ferred, brightly colored stickers and trinkets can be highly motivating. The sequential processing problems also argue for more holistic teaching strategies than reinforc-ing steps in a sequential task analysis. One would expect that SMS children would benefit more from approaches based on modeling and participation with a visual presentation than from highly verbal based sequential instruction.

Behavioral Support

Virtually all people with SMS will need significant behavioral support as children and adults. A functional behavioral analysis from a behavioral analyst familiar with the SMS phenotype is crucial in developing behavioral supports that are appropri-ate. Given the sometimes florid behavioral presentation of self-injury it is noteworthy that there have been no controlled behavioral studies that have examined the treat-ment of self-injury in SMS. There are, however, many features of the SMS phenotype that can be used to develop functional behavioral hypotheses and aid in the deter-mination of behavioral contributory and trigger events.

The sleep disorder must be viewed as a contributing factor in the behavioral prob-lems experienced by people with SMS. A sleep chart should always be kept and in many cases a sleep study at a sleep clinic should be considered. If the sleep distur-bance can be controlled in the ways previously mentioned, behavioral interventions should have a higher probability of success. The visual and auditory deficits associ-ated with SMS must also be viewed as contributory factors. Uncorrected vision or hearing should be investigated. The high incidence of otitis media should also be examined as a SIB factor. Finger/toe nail picking and yanking should be viewed in the context of peripheral neuropathy. Clinically, nail polish has been used success-fully to decrease this behavior.

Sequential processing and attention deficits should be examined as contributing to observed problem behavior. Again, the use of visuals, favored activities interspersed with less favored with clear simple instructions is the best way to structure the time of an individual with SMS. For individuals with expressive language problems, a communication system based on visuals is a must. Picture schedules and picture exchange systems can be of enormous help in aiding an individual to communicate with others and avoiding behavioral incidents that result from an inability to com-municate wants and needs. Behavioral interventions should include these components.

In settings where there are caregivers and multiple recipients, the fewer recipients present, the less likely it is that a problem behavior will develop. This is most often due to competition for attention from peers. For individuals with SMS in such living or vocational settings the extent that competition for caregiver attention contributes to the problem behavior should be assessed. The propensity to hug has also been implicated in some problem situations. There are reports of SMS individuals killing small pets. When investigated, these instances were due to the pets being "hugged to death" as the SMS individual displayed their excitement and happiness.

The best way to behaviorally treat an individual with SMS is to make use of syndromic strengths and weaknesses as an aid to developing a behavioral support plan that minimizes contributory factors and maximizes strengths. Even in a SMS "friendly" environment that takes into account biological and behavioral profiles there is apt to be some instances of SIB and tantrums. In these instances it is important to intervene as early as possible. It is often easy to tell that a person with SMS is escalating their behavior to the "point of no return" and that a tantrum will occur. If the behavioral course can be addressed before the tantrum escalates, there is often a good chance that the full-blown tantrum can be avoided. Clinically, I have found that when a person with SMS begins a tantrum sequence, a tantrum can be avoided by redirecting the individual to a quiet one-on-one conversation on a topic that the individual likes, or engaging the individual in a preferred activity with one on one attention. This is sometimes difficult to do as it may be seen as rewarding the escalating behavior. However, it appears to serve a calming function and fill the need for attention that in most cases was the trigger for the behavioral escalation in the first place. In a few minutes time the individual can be redirected back to the original situation without incident.

There will also, of course be times where a major tantrum cannot be avoided. In these instances it is best to withdraw attention and let the person know that you will be there for them when they are ready to interact with you. Removing the individual from the environment where the tantrum has begun, if possible, can sometimes aid the dissolution of the behavior. This may be due to the people who were competing for attention in the first place no longer being present and able to be viewed in that way.

Psychopharmacological

Prescribing psychotropic medications based on successful use in a particular genetic syndrome is a controversial topic, and clearly no individual with SMS should be prescribed a medication simply because they have been diagnosed with SMS. However, as the behavioral profiles of individuals with SMS can include attentional problems, hyperactivity, self-injury, aggression, sleep disorder and mood lability, psychotropic medications are often in use. If an individual with SMS meets the DSM IV (1994) criteria for a known psychiatric disorder, then medication appropriate for that disorder should be considered. In the future, knowledge of which psychiatric disorders are more prevalent and which medications have been most successful in treating these disorders in SMS individuals will aid in deciding on an appropriate medication. There are, however, no controlled studies of medication use in SMS to date, reports of medication usage are based on clinical experience with small numbers of individuals.

As previously stated, many individuals with SMS meet the criteria for attention deficit disorder with or without hyperactivity. Hagerman (1999a; 1999b) reports that there is anecdotal evidence that the stimulants methylphenidate, adderall, and dextroamphetamine can positively affect theses symptoms (Allen, 1998, cited in Hagerman, 1999a).

Given the mood swings and sleep disorder that is present, individuals with SMS also can meet the criteria for bipolar disorder. The SSRI medications have been suggested as effectively treating these mood swings (Smith & Gropman, 2001). Greenberg et al. (1996) recommends that the anticonvulsant mood stabilizers carbamazepine or valproic acid be tried in these instances. Hagerman (1999a) also suggests that risperidone has been used with some success.

I have observed that adults with SMS respond well to a cojoint approach of behavioral support and medication usage. We have utilized a protocol of carbamazepine augmented with risperidone. Initially, risperidone has been necessary to stabilize the individual while titrating the mood stabilizer to a level in the high therapeutic range. For adults, once the mood stabilizer reaches acceptable levels, we have been able to decrease the risperidone to a dosage of 1 to 2 mgs.

Family Support

Families with a member who has SMS are clearly under increased stress. Although supporting any individual with a developmental disability is stressful for the family, the severe behavioral presentation of SMS can be particularly stressful. Parents of children with SMS report sleeping in shifts to ensure their child's safety. Hodapp, Fidler, and Smith (1998) have examined the stress and coping in 41 families of children with SMS using standardized assessments of stress and behavior. High levels of both stress and family support were found, with the size of the family support system the best overall predictor of family stress. The more family friends and the larger number of individuals in the family support circle, the lower the stress. Families made use of professional support to a great degree, with 76% reporting a professional in their family support circle.

Given these results, the use of outside family support services such as friends and professionals is very important for the overall welfare of the family. Participation in the national support group PRISMS should be recommended to all families. PRISMS can be contacted at 76 South New Boston Road, Francestown, NH 03043-3511. There is also a national conference sponsored by PRISMS. Information on the national conference and the many other services available through this organization is available from PRISMS or on their Internet Web site: www.smithmagenis.org.

With the advent of the World Wide Web, many families are supporting each other through the use of listservs. A listserv allows individuals interested in a specific topic to sign up to receive e-mail that is directed to a list address. Given the rarity of many genetic disorders, a listserv is the perfect opportunity for families of children with specific genetic disorders to network and meet each other, compare experiences and support each other. SMS has a particularly active listserv that has been in existence since 1998. There are typically over 100 messages per month from family members and professionals. Monthly messages are archived and can be easily accessed. To join the SMS online discussion or to view the archived messages go to the following World Wide Web address: http://groups.yahoo.com/group/sms-list/.

Summary and Conclusions

The SMS is a clearly defined genetic syndrome with characteristic behavioral, psychological, medical and physical features. These features affect the way individuals processes information, react to the environment and are perceived by those around them. It is becoming apparent that there are specific developmental pathways to these features. As these pathways become elucidated, clinicians and support staff will be better able to incorporate them into educative and life support strategies. There already exist several recommendations for the support of individuals with SMS with regard to medical service, classroom structuring and teaching strategies. Using the underlying physical and medical characteristics of the syndrome by psychologists and behavioral analysts appears particularly promising. Likewise, treatment and support for all disciplines will increasingly adopt a conceptualization that is based on an etiological SMS orientation. As this occurs, staff will view themselves as supporting an individual with SMS, as opposed to the current widespread approach, that plans for the needs of an individual with mental retardation who has disparate strengths and needs in a variety of areas. As progress is made in understanding the underlying biochemical pathways from chromosome deletion to expressed behavior, medical and physical characteristics, supports and treatment will increasingly take on this biopsychosocial cohesive syndromic approach.

Resources

The following resources are available to families and professionals interested in the SMS. They are taken from PRISMS recommendations:

Parents and Researchers Interested in Smith Magenis Syndrome, 76 South New Boston Road, Francestown, NH 03043-3511 www.smithmagenis.org

Smith Magenis Contact Group (U.K.) , 1 Poppyfields Chester-le-Street, Co. Durham, DH2 2NA England, UK

Online Mendelian Inheritance in Man-SMS entry: http:// www3.ncbi.nlm.nih.gov/htbin-post/Omim/dispmim?182290

ASM-17 Association Smith Magenis (France)- http://membres.lycos.fr/ asm17france/

Baylor School of Medicine SMS Project- Lorraine Potocki, M.D. or James R. Lupski, M.D., Ph.D. Department of Molecular and Human Genetics Baylor College of Medicine, One Baylor Plaza, Room 609E, Houston, TX 77030

The Smith Magenis Listserv, http://groups.yahoo.com/group/sms-list/

Elwyn Inc. Genetic Outreach , SMS Consultation and Technical Assistance to Schools and Adult Support Teams, Brenda Finucane, M.S., Elwyn Inc., 111 Elwyn Road, Elwyn, PA 19063.

The National Human Genome Research Institute Smith Magenis Protocol- to understand the behavioral and cognitive characteristics of SMS with special attention to life span development. Contact: Ann CM Smith, MS, DSc (hon) Head, SMS Research Unit, National Human Genome Research Institute, National Institutes of Health, 9000 Rockville Pike, Bethesda, MD 20892-2152, or E-mail: acsmith@nhgri.nih.gov

References

American Psychiatric Association. (1987). *Diagnostic and statistical manual of mental disorders* (3rd ed., revised). Washington, DC: Author.

American Psychiatric Association. (1994). *Diagnostic and statistical manual of mental disorders* (4th ed.). Washington, DC: Author.

Chen, K. S., Lupski, J. R., Greenberg, F., & Lewis, R. A. (1996). Opthalmic manifestations of Smith–Magenis syndrome. *Opthalmology, 103*, 1084-1091.

Colley, A. F., Leversha, M. F., Voullaire, L. E., & Rogers, J. G. (1990). Five cases demonstrating the distinctive features of chromosome deletion 17(p11.2 p11.2) Smith-Magenis syndrome). *Journal of Pediatric Child Health, 26*, 17-24.

DeLeersnyder, H. & Munnich, A. (1999). Abnormal sleep patterns and behavioral difficulties in patients with Smith-Magenis Syndrome are due to an inversion in the circadian rhythm of melatonin. Paper presented at the 49th Annual Meeting of the American Society of Human Genetics, San Francisco, CA, October 1999.

Dykens, E. M., Finucane, B. M. , & Gayley, C. (1997). Brief report: Cognitive and behavioral profiles in persons with Smith-Magenis Syndrome. *Journal of Autism and Developmental Disorders, 27,* 203-211.

Dykens, E., & Smith, A. C. (1998). Distinctiveness and correlates of maladaptive behavior in children and adults with Smith-Magenis syndrome. *Journal of Intellectual Disability Research, 42*, 481-489.

Finucane, B., Dirrigl, K. H. and Simon, E. W. (2001). Characterization of self-injurious behaviors in children and adults with Smith-Magenis syndrome. *American Journal of Mental Retardation , 106*, 52-58.

Finucane, B. M., Konar, D., Haas-Givler, B., & Kurtz, M. B. (1994). The spasmodic upper body squeeze: a characteristic behavior in Smith-Magenis syndrome. *Developmental Medicine and Child Neurology, 36*, 78-83.

Finucane, B. M., Jaeger E. R., Kurtz, M. B., Weinstein, M., & Scott C. I. (1993). Eye abnormalities in the Smith-Magenis contiguous gene deletion syndrome. *American Journal of Medical Genetics, 45*, 443-446.

Finucane, B., & Simon, E. W. (1999). Genetics and dual diagnosis: Smith-Magenis Syndrome. *The NADD Bulletin, 2*, 8-10.

GeneClinics (2002). Smith-Magenis Syndrome [del(17)(p11.2)], http://www.geneclinics.org.

Greenberg, F., Guzetta, V., De Oca-Luna, R. M., Magenis, R. E., Smith, A. C. M., Richter, S. F., et al. (1991). Molecular analysis of the Smith-Magenis syndrome: A possible contiguous-gene syndrome associated with del(17)(p11.2). *American Journal of Human Genetics, 49*, 1207-1218.

Greenberg, F., Lewis, R. A., Potocki, L., Glaze, D., Parke, J., Killian, J., Murphy, M. A., et al. (1996). Multi-disciplinary clinical study of Smith-Magenis syndrome (deletion 17p11.2). *American Journal of Medical Genetics, 62*, 247-254.

Haas-Givler, B. (1994). Educational implications and behavioral concerns of SMS: From the teacher's perspective. *Spectrum, 1*, 36-38.

Haas-Givler, B. (1996). Observations on the behavioral and personality characteristics of children with Smith-Magenis syndrome. *Genetwork, 2*, 4-5.

Haas-Givler, B., & Finucane, B. (1996). What's a teacher to do? Classroom strategies that enhance learning for children with SMS. *Genetwork, 2*, 6-10.

Hagerman, R. (1999a). Psychopharmacological interventions in fragile X syndrome, fetal alcohol syndrome, Prader-Willi syndrome, Angelman syndrome, Smith-Magenis syndrome, and velocardiofacial syndrome. *Mental Retardation and Developmental Disabilities Research Reviews, 5*, 305-313.

Hagerman, R. J. (1999b). Smith Magenis Syndrome. In R.J. Hagerman, *Neurodevelopmental Disorders: Diagnosis and Treatment* (pp.341-364). New York: Oxford University Press.

Hodapp, R. M., Fidler, D. J. & Smith, A. C. M. (1998). Stress and coping in families of children with Smith-Magenis syndrome. *Journal of Intellectual Disability Research, 42*, 331-340.

Kaufman, A. S., & Kaufman, N. L. (1984). *Kaufman Assessment Battery for Children.* Circle Pines MN: American Guidance Service.

Kaufman, A. S., & Kaufman, N. L. (1992). *Kaufman Assessment Battery for Adolescents and Adults.* Circle Pines, MN: American Guidance Service.

Lockwood, D., Hecht, F., Dowman, C., Hecht, B. K., Rizkallah, T. H., Goodwin, T. M. & Allanson, J. (1988). Chromosome subband 17p11.2 deletion: A minute deletion syndrome. *Journal of Medical Genetics, 25*, 732-737.

Reiss, S. (1988). *Reiss Screen for Maladaptive Behavior.* Chicago, IL: International Diagnostic Systems Inc.

Simon, E. W., & Finucane, B. (1998). Etiology and dual diagnosis: Notes on a biologically based syndromic approach. *The NADD Bulletin, 1,* 63-65.

Smith, A. C., Dykens, E., & Greenberg, F. (1998a). Behavioral phenotype of Smith-Magenis syndrome (del 17p11.2). *American Journal of Medical Genetics (Neuropsychiatric Genetics), 81,* 179-185.

Smith, A. C., Dykens, E., & Greenberg, F. (1998b). Sleep disturbance in Smith-Magenis syndrome. *American Journal of Medical Genetics, 81,* 186-191.

Smith, A. C., & Gropman (1999). Smith-Magenis Syndrome. In S. Cassidy, J. Allanson (Eds.), *Clinical management of common genetic syndromes (pp 363-387).* New York: John Wiley.

Smith, A. C. M., McGavran, L., Robinson, J., Waldstein, G., Macfarlane, J., Zonona, et al., (1986). Interstitial deletion of (17) (p.11.2) in nine patients. *American Journal of Medical Genetics, 24,* 421-432.

Vostanis, P., Harrington, R., Prendergast, M., & Farndon, P. (1994). Case reports of autism with interstitial deletion of chromosome 17 (p11.2 p11.2) and monosomy of chromosome 5 (5pter->5p15.3). *Psychiatric Genetics, 4,* 109-111.

Zori, R. T., Lupski, J. R., Heju, Z., Greenberg, F., Killian, J. M., Gray, B. A., et al., (1993). Clinical, cytogenetic, and molecular evidence for an infant with Smith-Magenis syndrome born from a mother having a mosaic 17p11.2p12 deletion. *American Journal of Medical Genetics, 47,* 504-511.

CHAPTER 6

Pervasive Developmental Disorders

Sandra Fisman

Introduction

Patrick is 4 years old. He has been referred to a multidisciplinary children's treatment center because of his unusual language and his lack of social development. His mother had sensed that "something was not right with Patrick" since his early infancy. He was content to be left alone in his crib, lacked social responsiveness and failed to make strange in his first year of life. He had shown a preference for carpet tassels, ignoring his toys as a toddler except to line them up in rows and spin the wheels on his toy trunk. Both parents questioned Patrick's hearing abilities at this time as he appeared to ignore them and did not respond to his name. However, other sounds such as the vacuum cleaner or lawn mower seemed very upsetting to him and he would cup his hands over his ears screaming at high pitch. Between age 2 and the present, Patrick increasingly became fascinated by letters and numbers. Patrick's motor milestones were all achieved on time. His language development (both expressive and receptive) had been quite delayed and his present language is largely composed of repetitive chunks and echoes. Patrick was proving very difficult to toilet train and insistent on having his bowel movement with a diaper on. Patrick has a diagnosis of autism.

Leo Kanner in 1943 and Hans Asperger in 1944 provided the descriptions of autism that are the basis for the current classification system in the Diagnostic and Statistical Manual (4ᵗʰ Edition) of the American Psychiatric Association (DSM-IV) (1994). However, descriptions of individuals akin to Kanner's autism date back to the late eighteenth century. Amongst these descriptions are feral children who were abandoned to the wild and recaptured into society. Itard, the savior of Victor the wild boy of Aveyron in France, provides us with a comprehensive case history that is strongly suggestive of autism. Itard's struggles to educate and socialize Victor, his frustrations and his joy with small accomplishments resonate for those who care for, teach, and train this hard to serve population. It is with these caretakers and professionals in mind that this chapter has been written.

Diagnostic Features

Diagnostic Misconceptions

Prior to 1980, when the Pervasive Developmental Disorders (PDDs) were first included as a separate category in the third edition of the American Psychiatric Association Diagnostic and Statistical Manual, autism was conceptualized as a form of childhood psychosis (Creak, 1963). This led to the lumping together of a heterogeneous group of children with impaired relating, abnormal perceptual sensitivities, poorly modulated anxiety, disordered language and a lack of sense of self.

Kanner's description of 11 children in his 1943 paper titled "Autistic Disturbances of Affective Contact" in the journal *Nervous Child* provided a durable account of classic autism. The triad of deficits in social relatedness, insistence on sameness, and language abnormalities continue to guide our diagnostic systems. However, Kanner provided some false research leads that delayed progress in this field. His use of the term "autism," borrowed from adult psychiatry, suggested that these children were part of an inclusive view of schizophrenia. This issue was only resolved in 1971 (Kolvin) when the differentiation of these children from individuals with schizophrenia was clearly established through emphasis on age of onset, clinical course, and family history.

A second false lead was in the area of cognition. Kanner believed that the "islets of ability" that he observed in these children, including phenomenal rote memory for names and rhymes and the recollection of complex patterns, sequences, and earlier events, bespoke above average intelligence. It took several decades to dispel this idea. The notion that some children with autism have preserved intellectual skills has persisted in spite of established evidence that the majority of autistic children score in the mentally retarded range on psychometric evaluation.

The third and final false lead has probably been the greatest source of heartbreak for the parents of these children. The idea that the cause of autism originated in problematic parent-child interactions where parents were high achieving, professional individuals, was congruent with the psychoanalytic ethos of the nineteen fifties and nineteen sixties. The term "refrigerator mother" encapsulates the essence of this idea. As controlled studies were conducted in the nineteen seventies clear evidence emerged that parents of autistic children were neither deficient in their care-giving (Cantwell, Rutter, & Baker, 1978) nor, as a group, did they present with higher levels of occupational and educational achievement.

Evolution of Diagnostic Concepts

It was not until 1980 that the PDDs were recognized as a distinct group of disorders separate from schizophrenia. In DSM-III autism was included under the umbrella of the PDDs. Criteria for the diagnosis of childhood schizophrenia were subsumed with the adult disorder (DSM-III) (American Psychiatric Association, 1980). In the DSM-III age of onset prior to or after 30 months of age (i.e., infantile autism versus childhood onset PDD) and the absence of delusions and hallucinations were recognized as important defining characteristics of this group of disorders.

The concept of an autistic spectrum, rather than age of onset, influenced the diagnostic criteria for PDD in the third, revised edition of the DSM—DSM-III-R (American Psychiatric Association, 1987). This concept evolved from an epidemiological survey of mentally and physically handicapped children conducted in Camberwell, a borough of inner London (Wing & Gould, 1979). In the Camberwell study, social impairment was defined as an inability to engage in two-way social interaction. The quality of this impairment was captured in three distinct descriptors: aloof, passive, and active but odd. Accompanying the impaired two-way social interaction were abnormalities in verbal and non verbal communication and restricted interests carried out in a repetitive fashion. The three clusters of difficulty were referred to as the "autistic triad." It was acknowledged that children could have varying degrees of difficulties in these three areas. Those who showed abnormalities in all aspects of the triad were considered part of the autistic spectrum disorders (Wing,1981; 1986). It was suggested that Asperger's Disorder was at one end of the continuum and low functioning autism on the other. However, the DSM-III-R provided only two diagnostic options: autistic disorder representing classic Kanner's autism and the much broader category of Pervasive Developmental Disorder Not Otherwise Specified (PDD-NOS). This resulted in a classification system that was highly sensitive but low in specificity. (Volkmar, Cicchett, Bregman, & Cohen, 1992).

Current Diagnostic Concepts

In more recent years, evidence has accumulated to support a categorical approach to the diagnosis of the PDDs. This approach was reflected first in the 10th edition of the International Classification of Diseases—ICD (World Health Organization, 1990). It was subsequently repeated in the DSM-IV (American Psychiatric Association, 1994). Other categories grouped with autistic disorder in the PDD class include Asperger's Disorder, Rett's Disorder, Childhood Disintegrative Disorder, and Pervasive Developmental Disorder Not Otherwise Specified (PDD-NOS) (including Atypical Autism). The PDD-NOS category is used when criteria for one of the specific pervasive developmental disorders are not met but there is a severe and pervasive impairment of two way social interaction or of verbal and non-verbal communication or the presence of stereotyped behavior, interests and activities. The concept of the "autistic triad' of symptoms is maintained in DSM-IV. A brief description of each main PDD category follows.

Autistic Disorder

Autistic disorder is the paradigmatic PDD. A disturbance in social relatedness is the major defining feature of the disorder. Typically, this disorder has a very early age of onset; difficulties are most often noted in the first year of life but there may be a period of one or two years of apparently normal development prior to the onset of autistic symtomatology (Short & Schopler, 1988).

Children with autistic disorder have profound problems with all aspects of communication (verbal and non verbal) and language is both delayed and deviant (Frith, 1991). Many autistic individuals remain non-verbal and for those who develop speech, prolonged echolalia, pronoun reversal, unusual prosody and extreme literalness are typical. Approximately 20-30% of autistic individuals have IQs above the 70 cut off point— i.e., in the non-retarded range. However, high-functioning individuals whose IQ is within the normal range have considerable difficulty with the nuances of social language and recognition of non verbal cues. In addition, social adaptive behavior lags behind cognitive ability, adding to the child's functional impairment.

Autistic children display a range of unusual behaviors, which are captured in the overall descriptors of resistance to change or insistence on sameness. Children may insist on a particular routine, become very difficult during transitions and become preoccupied with objects or particular repetitive activities.

Mental retardation is associated with autism in at least 75% of cases (Lord & Rutter, 1994) and is the single most powerful predictor of outcome (Ventner, Lord, & Schopler., 1992). Children who do not have useful speech by late childhood show a decline in overall IQ (Waterhouse & Fein, 1997). The unevenness in intellectual profile with splinter ability in some tests of spatial ability such as block design and in rote memory skills suggest that impairment in a number of cognitive processes may be contributing to the overall lower IQ in these children (Sigman, Arbelle, & Dissanayake, 1995).

Asperger's Disorder

Asperger was a Viennese pediatrician who described a group of children with social isolation, pedantic speech, one-sided conversation with others and eccentric unusual interests that occupy a large part of their time. The disorder was said to be more common in boys than girls. Asperger believed that intelligence in these children was above average.

Although the differentiation of high functioning autism and Asperger's Disorder continues to be debated (Rutter & Schopler, 1992), there is support for separate categorization of these two disorders (Szatmari, Archer, Fisman, Streiner, & Wilson, 1995). In contrast to autistic disorder, there are no clinically significant delays in language, cognitive development or age-appropriate self help and adaptive skills (other than social interaction) in children with Asperger's Disorder. Diagnostic criteria also include the presence of significant functional impairment (social, occupational or both) (American Psychiatric Associaton, 1994). Differentiation between the two disorders has also been made in terms of neuropsychological abnormalities: Asperger's Disorder is often associated with the psychometric profile of a Non-Verbal Learning Disability and underlying right hemispheric dysfunction (Rourke, 1989; Ellis, Ellis, Fraser, & Deb, 1994). Related to right hemispheric dysfunction and a lack of social awareness, may be an abnormality in "social gaze response" (Tantum, 1991). The failure to attend to faces of others suggests that these children do not learn about facial expressions and they miss cues that signal nonverbal information in the eye gaze of others.

Some investigators maintain that Asperger's Disorder is a mild variant of autism (Green, 1990). They argue that differentiation should be made between higher functioning and lower functioning individuals with lower functioning individuals with autism having more evidence of brain pathology and dysfunction and high functioning individuals with autism and Asperger's Disorder sharing similar underlying genetic abnormalities (DeLong & Dwyer, 1988). Also at issue, is the change over time in clinical presentation of the high functioning group. Gillberg (1991) has suggested that over time, high functioning autism comes to resemble Asperger's Disorder in terms of odd and eccentric interactions with others.

Rett's Disorder and Childhood Disintegrative Disorder

These disorders have been grouped with the PDDs because of the abnormalities of function that develop in the areas of social interaction, communication and stereotyped behaviors. Children with both disorders share a period of apparently normal development (for at least 5 months in the case of Rett's Disorder and at least 2 years with Childhood Disintegrative Disorder). Both disorders are typically associated with severe mental retardation and often follow a deteriorating course. While all of the other PDDs are more common in males, Rett's Disorder has only been reported in females. Characteristic of Rett's Disorder is the development of stereotyped hand movements resembling hand writing or hand washing, deceleration of head growth, and deterioration in gait. The ability to interact socially is lost early in the course of deterioration but there may be some recovery of this skill later.

Diagnostic Dilemmas

While diagnostic criteria, applied more consistently over recent years, have allowed us to more accurately categorize the PDDs, there remain a group of diagnostically confusing individuals whose presentation includes overlapping criteria for both the developmental language disorders and the PDDs.

In addition to the sensitivity and specificity for the PDD diagnostic categories, the clinical picture changes with age particularly in higher functioning and more verbal individuals. As a result, the clinician may have difficulty with diagnostic categorization on the one hand and on the other hand, the diagnostic picture may alter with development. These children have been labelled "semantic pragmatic disorder " (Bishop, 1989). As a group these children "shade into autism at one extreme and normality at the other" (Brook & Bowler, 1992). These and other diagnostic relationships and overlaps are represented graphically in the following diagram.

Overlap of PDD Diagnostic Categories and Developmental Language Disorders

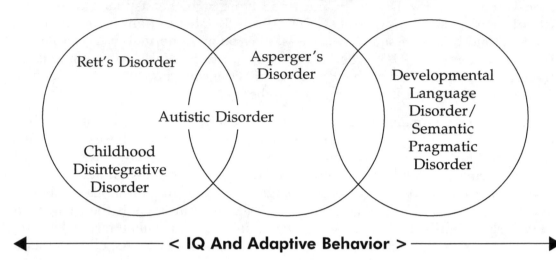

Rett's Disorder

Asperger's Disorder

Developmental Language Disorder/ Semantic Pragmatic Disorder

Autistic Disorder

Childhood Disintegrative Disorder

◄──────────── < IQ And Adaptive Behavior > ──────────►

The Neurobiology of the Pervasive Developmental Disorders

It is not surprising, given the heterogeneous clinical presentation of the PDDs, to discover that diverse mechanisms of central nervous system dysfunction have been implicated in the etiology of these disorders. Ideally this diversity should reflect the diagnostic categories that we have reviewed. However, our current state of knowledge reflects descriptive phenomenology of these disorders rather than a precise understanding of their pathogenesis. A parallel example would be the case of epilepsy or cerebral palsy where there is neurologic dysfunction but the specific etiology and pathogenesis varies from case to case.

Although the specific abnormalities of brain function in the PDDs remain elusive, there have been considerable advances in the genetic and neuropsychological studies of these disorders. Increasingly sophisticated neuroimaging techniques and neurochemical studies are also adding to our understanding of these disorders, providing some rationale for biological treatments, specifically pharmacotherapy. Each of these areas will be briefly reviewed.

Genetic Considerations

At the present time autism and its related disorders are thought to have high heritability. However, this has not always been the case. Although Kanner postulated in his initial description of autism that it was an inborn disorder, the prevalent opinion until recently was that there was little evidence for a genetic etiology in autism. The current focus is not on autism as a genetic disorder but, rather, which specific genes and genetic mechanisms might be involved. The evidence for a strong genetic basis for these disorders comes from twin and sibling studies particularly those studies of multiplex families where more than one child has a PDD disorder or a PDD variant.

There have been four general-population based twin studies of autism: two British studies (Folstein & Rutter, 1977; Bailey et al., 1995), a Norwegian study (Steffenburg et al., 1989) and a U.S. study in Utah (Ritvo, Spence, Freeman, Mason-Brothers, Mo, & Marazita, 1985). The concordance rate for monozygotic twins ranged from 64 to 98% and 0 to 38% for the dizygotic twin pairs.

Smalley et al. (1988) summarized six studies of sibling risk for autism and estimated the risk to be 2.7%. In a population study of autism in Utah, Ritvo, et al. (1989) reported a sibling risk of 4.5% and a recurrence risk of 8.5% in a family. This higher risk for siblings in the Utah study may be explained by the presence of a large Mormon population in Utah who are not deterred from having further children after the birth of a child with a developmental disability. There is a tendency for parents with children who have early onset burdensome conditions to not have any further children. This stoppage effect, evidenced by the tendency for children with autism to be born late in their sibships or to be only children, may explain the above discrepant sibling risk figures. Even if the true risk for siblings was only 1%, this would still increase their risk, compared to the general population by as much as 25 times (Jones & Szatmari, 1988).

Variable Expressivity

In addition to the heritability risk for full-blown autistic disorder, the genes for autism may also result in susceptability to milder or incomplete manifestations of PDD. A spectrum of disorder is seen in first-degree relatives of children with PDD that ranges from Asperger's Disorder and atypical autism to a lesser variant of PDD. In the PDD lesser variant impairments in reciprocal social interaction, communication and interests may be insufficient to merit a PDD diagnosis.

The overall risk for PDDs to the siblings of PDD probands is 5-6% (Szatmari, Jones, Tuff, Bartolucci, Fisman, & Mahoney, 1993) while the risk for the lesser variant PDD is much higher. Bolton et al. (1994) found that 20% of siblings of autistic probands had social or communication impairments or a restricted pattern of interests compared to 3% of Down syndrome (DS) control siblings. Piven et al. (1994) reported that parents of autistic children were often rated as more aloof, tactless and unresponsive on a standardized personality interview than parents of DS controls. The lesser variant PDD has also been found in second and third degree relatives of PDD probands, suggesting that biological rather than environmental factors are operative in the family patterns of PDD transmission (Pickles et al., 1995).

What Is Inherited?

Genetic research supports that the PDDs are a heterogeneous group of disorders. This heterogeneity refers to the possibility that both genetic and environmental factors may contribute to the disorder (etiological heterogeneity) as well as the possibility that the PDDs may be caused by different genetic mechanisms (genetic heterogeneity).

There is good evidence for both genetic and etiological heterogeneity in the PDDs. As an example, autism can be associated with several known genetic disorders (e.g., Fragile X syndrome, tuberous sclerosis, neurofibromatosis and phenylketonuria). It can also be associated with congenital syndromes caused by the rubella and cytomegalovirus.

Six Rules for Genetic Counseling in PDD Families

1. A careful diagnostic assessment is an important start to confirm the diagnosis and rule out associated conditions.
2. Explanation of the relative risk for autism to family members in positive terms, e.g., a 19 out of 20 chance that a future child will not be autistic rather than a 1 in 20 chance the child will be.
3. There is significantly increased risk for the offspring if both parents have definite cases of autism in the family.
4. The risk for offspring of non-affected siblings is probably less than 1 in 500.
5. The risk for lesser variant symptoms in siblings is in the region of 10-20% but it should be emphasized that these individuals generally become self-sufficient adults.
6. It is not the task of the counselor to make decisions for the family but rather to facilitate the best available risk analysis in an empathic clinical context.

Do We Understand the Neurocognitive Deficits in the PDDs?

Individuals with autism may have weak central coherence. This means that they tend to process information in individual parts rather than in a context (Bailey, Phillips, & Rutter, 1996). Other neurocognitive theories have involved deficits in theory of mind and executive function paradigms.

Theory of mind is described as the capacity to attribute thoughts, feelings and desires to oneself and other people (Baron-Cohen, 1989). This theory distinguishes between first order thinking ("he thinks that...") and second order thinking ("he thinks that she thinks that ..."). Developmentally normal children master first order tasks by age seven. It is hypothesized that the lack of social reciprocity and communication failure in autism arises in the context of an inability to understand intentions and beliefs of others. Deficits compatible with theory of mind deficits have been found in 80% of verbal children with autism.

The most consistent finding in neuropsychological studies of people with high functioning PDD is an **abnormality of executive function.** This leads to problems with planning, sequencing, impulse control and attention. The prefrontal cortex of the brain plays an important role in these functions. This region of the brain is also involved in novel goal directed behavior and speech. Ozonoff and McEvoy (1994) suggest that tests of executive function such as the Wisconsin Card Sort test and The Tower of Hanoi demonstrate perseveration, difficulty shifting cognitive set, poor planning and deficits in working memory in individuals with autism.

Neuroanatomical Changes: Are There Structural Abnormalities in the Brain?

Neuroanatomical changes in autism and Asperger's Disorder have primarily been described in the prefrontal cortex, the thalamus, the temporal lobe, and the cerebellum. Findings are inconsistent due to different methods of imaging and small numbers of hetereogenous subjects.

Table 1: How Is the Brain Imaged?

Technique	How It Works	Brain Structure Measured	Brain Function Measured
Computer analysis of electroencephalogram (**EEG**)	Brain mapping by computer analysis of EEG		X
Computerized axial tomography (**CAT**)	Computer construction of x-ray images	X	
Positron emission tomography (**PET**)	Images radioactively labeled substances in the brain injected intravenously		X*
Single-photon-emission computed tomography (**SPECT**)	Images radioactively labeled substances in the brain injected intravenously or inhaled		X**
Magnetic Resonance Imaging (**MRI**)	Images molecular changes in brain cells exposed to a strong magnetic field; non-invasive.	X	X

*   *Measures regional brain blood flow, glucose utilization, neurochemical activity*
**   *Measures regional brain blood flow*

One of the most consistent neuroanatomic findings in individuals with autism has been an increase in brain volume (Piven, Arndt, Bailey, Havercamp, Andreasen, & Palmer, 1995). This was confirmed in an autopsy study which demonstrated a 100 to 200 gram increase in brain weight in individuals with autism (Bailey, Luthert, Bolton, Le Couteur, Rutter, & Harding, 1993).

In a SPECT study Zilbovicius et al. (1995) found lower frontal regional cerebral blood flow at age 3 years in autistic subjects as compared to controls. This normalized at age 6 years. This may indicate delayed frontal maturation in autism consistent with the frontal lobe cognitive findings that have been described.

The thalamus is a subcortical brain center that acts as a sensory or attentional filter to higher cortical centres including the prefrontal cortex. It is possible that abnormal frontal cortical development in PDD may be the result of an early thalamic lesion. Szelazek et al. (2000) have found decreased prefrontal activity and increased thalamic activity using functional MRI in Asperger subjects compared with their control siblings. Early thalamic-cortical dysfunction may also explain abnormalities in brain hemipheric lateralization that have been described in autism (Cantor, Thatcher, Hrybyk, & Kaye, 1986) and Asperger's Disorder (Semrud-Clikeman & Hynd, 1990).

The temporal lobe of the brain is involved in the control of language and memory. It has important connections with the limbic system that is involved in emotion and motivation and has connections with the frontal lobe. Using SPECT, Gillberg et al (1993) found decreased blood flow in the temporal lobes of high functioning autistic individuals.

Changes have been found in the cerebellum in imaging and post mortem studies. The cerebellum is associated with functions such as the conscious control of fine motor movement, speech and calculations. Study results have been very variable. Piven et al. (1997) have suggested that any increase in volume of the cerebellum is similar to the increased volume of the temporal, occipital and parietal lobes.

How About Neurochemical Changes?

Neurotransmitter changes have been described in individuals with autism. Neurotransmitters are best described as specialized chemical messengers that are synthesized and secreted by neurons to communicate with other neurons. Among the numerous excitatory and inhibitory neurotransmitters in the nervous system, serotonin and dopamine have been implicated in autism.

The most consistent findings have been in the serotonin system with elevated whole blood serotonin being the most consistent biological marker described to date (Martineau, Barthelemy, Jouve, Muh, & Lelord, 1992). Hyperserotonemia segregates in families; the presence of a hyperserotonemic autistic child has been related to a 2.5 fold increase in the likelihood of a hyperserotonemic relative (Leventhal, Cook, Morford, Ravitz, & Freedman, 1990). Medications affecting the serotonin system which have been used in the PDDs include serotonin agonists (clomipramine, paroxetine, citalopram, fluoxetine, fluvoxamine, sertraline, buspirone and fenfluramine) as well as serotonin antagonists (risperidone, olanzapine, quetiapine and clozapine).

An increase in the metabolite of dopamine (homovanillic acid – HVA) has been found in autistic children when compared with controls (Barthelemy et al., 1988; Gillberg & Svennoholm, 1987). Increased HVA levels seem to correlate with neurological impairment rather than a diagnosis of autism (Hameury et al., 1995). Controlled studies of medications which antagonize dopamine have been found to improve some of the behavioral symptoms of PDD including hyperactivity, aggression, temper tantrums, stereotypies and lack of social relatedness. Dopamine antagonists include haloperidol, pimozide, risperidone, olanzapine and clozapine. Drugs which are dopamine agonists such as amphetamines may worsen preexisting symptoms in children with autism.

Significant abnormalities in norepinephrine and epinephrine levels and their metabolites have not been found in the PDDs but some medications which decrease activity of the sympathetic nervous system may have a limited role in the treatment of PDD. These include propranolol and nadolol as well as clonidine.

Excessive brain opioid activity resulting in increased endorphins could account for some of the symptoms seen in autistic disorder including social deficits and decreased pain sensitivity (Panksepp & Sahley, 1987). However, studies of endorphin levels have been very variable and the response of individuals with autism to naltrexone, an opioid antagonist has been equally variable.

The Diagnostic and Assessment Process

Because of their unique and often uneven developmental profiles and behavioral difficulties, children with autism and other PDDs present a challenge to examiners and to their families. However, the interdisciplinary assessment of cognitive, social, communication and adaptive behavior skills are essential for planning intervention. A comprehensive initial assessment (see table 2) will provide a profile of the child's strength's and weaknesses. Intervention using a goal-focused approach that facilitates adaptation and minimizes interfering behaviors will then flow from the assessment process.

Important Issues to Consider in the Assessment Process

♦ **A developmental perspective** is essential in the assessment in order to interpret cognitive and adaptive functioning in relation to normative expectations for the age of the child. The tests that are chosen should be developmentally appropriate and be able to maximize the sampling of a wide-range of the child's skills. For example using a cognitive test that is heavily dependent on language will skew the assessment results in a non-verbal child with non-verbal intellectual ability. A measure of non-verbal intellectual ability using a test such as the Leiter International Performance Scale (Leiter, 1948) will provide a more accurate measure of the child's developmental profile and will better guide intervention strategies.

♦ **Understanding delays and deviance** in the child's developmental profile will provide a more accurate profile from which to plan interventions. **Delays** will be identified using standardized instruments of intellectual functioning combined with measures of adaptive behavior.

Information regarding **deviant behaviors** may be obtained from diagnostic instruments such as the Autism Diagnostic Interview-Revised (ADI-R) (Lord, Rutter, & Le Couteur,, 1994) or the use of the Autism Diagnostic Observation Schedule (ADOS) (Lord et al., 1989). These instruments are administered in a semi-structured fashion. The ADI-R focus' on parents' descriptions of their child's behavior in multiple areas. It assists the diagnostic process and provides relevant information about the child's developmental and behavioral history, current difficulties in social, communicative and behavioral areas and the parents' perception of the child's behavior and difficulties. The ADI-R has excellent validity and reliability and is a useful clinical as well as a research tool. As the name implies the ADOS is used to observe the child's communicative and social behaviors. The ADOS was developed for children who had a mental age of at least 3 years. A prelinguistic form of the instrument, PL-ADOS, has been developed.

♦ **Establishing the variability of the child's skills profile** provides a better assessment of the child's capacity for learning and adaptation than simply focussing on the numerical results of standardized assessment. There are two antithetical issues to consider: first of all it is important to delineate the child's strengths and deficits in the context of very variable test scores. Secondly, there should not be an expectation of generalization of ability from one exceptional splinter skill. For example, the precocious ability to recognize letters and words may not correlate with the ability to combine these letters into words and sentences, with reading comprehension or with the use of these words for the purpose of communication. Similarly, an unusual ability with number computation may not transfer to the understanding of basic money concepts such as making change. On the other hand the child's assets and strengths can be used to maximize his/her learning potential and optimize the learning environment.

♦ **Developing an inventory of functional skills** will provide an understanding of the child's everyday adaptation and response to real life demands. Use of a structured interview such as the Vineland Adaptive Behavior Scales (Sparrow, Balla, & Cicchetti, 1984) with the child's caregivers will provide standard scores, percentiles and age equivalents for adaptive behavior, communication, socialization, daily living and motor skills. The assessment information can then be used to inform program planning.

Table 2: Overview of the Initial Assessment

History of presenting difficulties

- Communication/imagination/play
- Social reciprocity
- Behavior
- Developmental history
- Pregnancy/delivery/neonatal period
- Social emotional development
  - Infant temperament/early attachment
  - Eye contact
  - Social smiling/anticipatory gestures
  - Stranger/separation anxiety
  - Development of relationships
- Language development
  - Prelanguage skills
  - Intent to communicate
  - Expressive/receptive language milestones
  - Deviant language— e.g., echolalia, pronoun reversal
  - Development of play skills
- Motor development
- Skill development
- General medical history and physical examination
- Baseline physical parameters
- Gross and fine motor coordination
- Family history
- Developmental disabilities/psychiatric illness
- Family coping/support
- Sibling adjustment
- Observational interview of child
- Mental status examination
- Relatedness
- Separation behavior

Ancillary tests/information

- Preschool/school report
- Psychological evaluation
- Cognitive testing using a nonverbal measure if indicated— e.g., Leiter International Performance Scale
- Measure of adaptive behavior— e.g., Vineland Adaptive Behavior Scale
- Speech/language evaluation
- Occupational therapy assessment when indicated for skill assessment
- Other consultations— e.g., Pediatrics, Neurology when indicated.

The Child with PDD in the Context of the Family

High levels of stress exist in both mothers and fathers in families with a child with PDD. While both experience parenting stress generated by the child's handicap, it is mothers rather than fathers who suffer from depression This depression correlates with their parenting distress (Wolf, Noh, Fisman, & Speechley, 1989).

Comparing the parents of children with PDD with parents who have a child with Down syndrome, both mothers and fathers of children with PDD described high levels of stress related to the decreased adaptability of their child (making parenting difficult because of the child's difficulty in adjusting to environmental change) increased demandingness (related to the frequency and severity of behavior problems); and decreased acceptability (perceiving their child as less attractive, less appropriate and less intelligent than desired). Parents of children with Down syndrome experienced an extra burden only in their child's acceptability (Noh, Dumas, Wolf, & Fisman, 1989).

In addition to the stress generated by the child with PDD, the mothers (and not the fathers) experience additional parental stress related to their own feelings of dysphoria, a sense of lack of competence in parenting and feelings of poor health. There is a spill over into the marital relationship (Fisman, Wolf, & Noh, 1989) with mothers of children with PDD experiencing lowered levels of marital intimacy. This relates to a lowered sense of spousal self-esteem and a lack of recreation time in the marriage.

The emotional and behavioral adjustment of the unaffected siblings of children with PDD also shows an impact. Once again, it is the high level of parenting stress that impacts sibling adjustment (Fisman, Wolf, Ellison, & Freeman, 2000). In addition, those factors that are normally protective for children in families such as marital satisfaction, lack of parental depression, a cohesive family and a warm, nonconflictual sibling relationship do not appear to be operative for siblings in these highly stressed families (Fisman, Wolf, Ellison, Gillis, Freeman, & Szatmari, 1996). Because of the demands of the very difficult child with PDD the nondisabled sibling may feel neglected and their needs ignored. This is reflected in the tendency for unaffected siblings to externalize their distress with behavior problems at a younger age and to develop more internalizing symptoms (anxiety and depression) with the transition into puberty (Wolf, Fisman, & Ellison, 1998).

The question has been raised that there may be an increased rate of mood and anxiety disorders in the parents and siblings of children with autism apart from the stress factor (Smalley, McCracken, & Tanguay, 1995). However, none of the twin studies has confirmed this and a family history study (Szatmari et al., 1995) did not find that the rates of psychiatric symptoms were increased in extended relatives compared with controls.

The impact of living with a child with PDD and the effect on the entire family system has implications for planning interventions. While parents and siblings need to become partners in treatment, this cannot be done without consideration of the needs of unaffected family members both for considerable formal as well as informal support.

Effective Intervention Strategies in Pervasive Developmental Disorders Across the Lifespan

With the rejection of the final remnants of the self-blame hypothesis and the acceptance that these disorders are biologically based, the field of intervention has been able to move forward over the past two decades. The main goals for intervention at every phase of the life cycle are to optimize skill development and adaptation, especially language and social skills, and to minimize interfering behaviors particularly aggression and self-harm. A range of biological, structured social and behavioral interventions have been developed. Treatment planning needs to take place in the context of the family system with an awareness of the need for social support to nondisabled family members and an appreciation of what is possible in the individual family context. Consideration must be given to effective educational and community interventions. With the transition to adulthood there is necessarily a shift from predominantly family to predominantly community-based supports.

Early Intervention and Applied Behavioral Analysis (ABA)

The application of the rules by which behavior is determined by environmental factors to improve socially important behaviors is referred to as applied behavioral analysis. Applying these principles in the early years with children who have PDD may alter their developmental trajectory.

Lovaas (1987) described dramatic improvements with his early intervention program. Harris and Handleman (1994) have described the factors that characterize **effective** early **intervention programs**. These include:

- Individualized comprehensive programming
- Assessment of the child's strengths and deficits
- Identification of contextual variables that affect the child's behavior
- Linking assessment findings to curriculum
- Favorable teacher to child ratios, including one-to-one in the early stages of programming and interaction with peers in the child with PDD's natural environment.

Overview of Intervention Approaches

Behavioral Interventions

Behavioral interventions can be divided into three broad categories: a) those that target antecedents to a particular behavior; b) those that consequence a particular behavior; and c) those that promote skill development. In all categories the planned treatment intervention is based on a thorough functional analysis of behavior and skills.

Antecedent interventions are implemented **before** the expected target behaviors occur. These may be useful across the life span in reducing problem behaviors. For example, environmental changes that reduce visual distractions can result in a decrease in self-stimulatorybehavior in adolescents and adults with autism.

Consequence-based interventions are procedures that are implemented **as a result of** a problem behavior. Consequence based interventions are most effectively used when combined in a "package" with antecedent and skill building interventions. See Table 3.

Table 3: Most Frequently Used Consequence-based Interventions

Interruption and Redirection	Physical prevention of an undesirable behavior and redirection to an alternative acceptable activity
Reinforcement-Based Procedures	Use of a response to a desirable behavior to increase its future occurrence
Extinction Procedures	Withholding a response to reduce the occurrence of an undesirable behavior
Punishment Procedures	A response that decreases the future occurrence of an undesirable behavior

In using **consequence based interventions** the reinforcer must be powerful enough to motivate the individual to carry out a targeted desirable behavior. Interviews with caregivers and teachers and observational techniques are necessary to identify reinforcers (Mason, McGee, Farmer-Dougan, & Risley, 1989). Cautious and judicious use of the problem behavior— e.g., self-stimulation may be used for very brief periods to reinforce appropriate behavior. Extinction procedures are time consuming, do not, on their own, lead to alternative appropriate behavior development, and may result in a transient increase in the behavior.

Punishment procedures remain controversial but when used they may be more effective with systematic variation over time e.g., verbal reprimand, over-correction and time out applied in a scheduled fashion to a behavior problem.

Skill acquisition is at the core of intervention for individuals with PDD. Skills not only improve functionality but also replace problem behaviors. Teaching new, adaptive skills is central to the development of successful educational programs. Skill acquisition programs fall into four main areas: **language and communication; social skills; self-help** and **self-management skills;** and **prevocational/vocational skills.**

The goals for language and communication therapy are to acquire socially meaningful speech and/or to develop functional communication skills that replace negative behavioral communication. These skills are best taught in naturalistic settings rather than in isolated environments. This has meant a shift from teaching rudimentary speech with reinforcement strategies unrelated to social communication to the reliance on inherent reinforcement in a social setting. For example, young children are taught with a variety of interesting toys relying on the reinforcement of the toys and the interaction between child and adult to stimulate communication. Similarly, adolescents can be taught the names of food items in the context of a functional activity such as meal preparation.

Functional communication training is also used for minimally verbal or nonverbal individuals. Gestures or signs can be used both for receptive purposes to supplement speech expressed by the caregiver and for expressive purposes by the PDD individual to make meaningful requests (Carr & Kemp, 1989). Augmentative devices have become invaluable for nonverbal people (Schuler, Prizant, & Wetherby, 1997). At their simplest this is a picture, symbol, or word board to which the individual can point. Their most elaborate form is a hand held electronic device (a memo writer) that provides a printed message or functions as a voice synthesizer.

Social skills deficits are central to the PDDs. They range from a total aloofness and absence of social engagement seen in some individuals with autistic disorder to a lack of social reciprocity and empathy for others in people with Asperger's Disorder.

Social skills training (see Table 4) can have a major impact in improving behavioral functioning across the life span for persons with PDD. This is a necessary component of any comprehensive intervention program. Much like functional communication, social skills are best taught in natural settings and in pairs or groups. Peer modeling is a useful strategy for teaching social skills. Classroom interventions using peer tutoring have been effective in improving social and academic skills of the child with PDD as well as normally developing classmates (Kamps, Barbetta, Leonard, & Delquadri, 1994). In addition to modeling by average peers and by the group leader, social skills groups utilize role-play of social interactions and rehearsal of behaviors to be used in the community.

Table 4: Components of a Social Skills Training Program

- Keeping appropriate physical distance
- Learning to initiate and terminate interactions
- Teaching flexibility in novel situations
- Voice modulation
- Recognizing and responding to emotions in others
- Understanding humor

Self-help skills training in the preschool and early school-age population and **self-management skills training** in the older child, adolescent and adult with PDD are designed to increase capacity for optimal independence. While these skills are acquired naturally in individuals without developmental disabilities, they must be taught painstakingly in persons with PDD.

The focus for self-help skills training in the preschool child will be in the areas of feeding, toileting, grooming and dressing as well as fine motor and gross motor coordination skills. In the older child and through to adulthood there is a shift to community awareness skills and introduction of self-management skills. The latter are behavioral strategies where persons take responsibility for their own behavior. Aids are generally used to help the individual self-monitor. Examples include pictorial or written schedules which break tasks down into component parts (Koegel, Koegel, Hurley, & Frea, 1992; Pierce & Shreibman, 1994). Both children and adults learn to administer their own contingent rewards and consequences.

Building provocational and vocational skills are a critical element in making the transition for PDD individuals from the educational system to the "real world." The opportunities to acquire these skills are best accomplished in a structured transition plan with clearly defined immediate and long-term goals coodinated by a case manager (Stowitzcheck, 1992). The entire transition plan needs to include leisure and living options in addition to an appropriate vocational plan. Prevocational skills training should begin in the educational curriculum with transportation training, money management training and social skills appropriate for the workplace.

Pharmacotherapy

Medication can be helpful for some individuals with PDD particularly where they are used in the context of a comprehensive treatment plan. There are two principles that guide the selection of a particular psychopharmalogic agent: The first relates the neurochemical action of the recommended medication to a **neurotransmittor system** that may be disordered as was described under neurobiology of the PDDs; the second guides medication choice by targeting the most interfering symptom(s). While the use of a single medication is preferable, sometimes it becomes necessary to combine agents to optimize the response to medication. A summary of the more commonly used medications, their neurochemical action(s) and target symptoms follows in Table 5.

Life Cycle Transitions

For the individual with PDD and his or her family the negotiation of developmental transitions is accentuated and complicated. As we have discussed, the burden of care-taking frequently falls on the mother but there is an impact on all family members. Life cycle transitions as they pertain to a family with a PDD member will be reviewed briefly with some suggestions for coping strategies.

The Crisis of Diagnosis

The crisis of diagnosis is associated with pain and grieving although parents, particularly the primary caretaker parent, and sometimes other close family members

Table 5: Action of Most Commonly Used Medications for PDD

MEDICATION	MAIN NEURO-CHEMICAL EFFECT	TARGET SYMPTOMS	MAIN DISADVANTAGE
Clomipramine	5-HT, NE, DA	Aggression, social relatedness, mood, repetitive behaviors, SIB.	May increase agitation/aggression. May lower seizure threshold.
Fluoxetine	5-HT	Social relatedness, transitions, mood, repetitive behaviors, SIB.	Restlessness/agitation, insomnia/decreased appetite.
Fluvoxamine	5-HT	Aggression, social relatedness, transitions, mood, repetitive behaviors, SIB.	Nausea/decreased appetite.
Sertraline	5-HT	Social relatedness, transitions, mood, repetitive behaviors, SIB.	Increased agitation, occasionally.
Buspirone	5–HT, DA	Aggression, mood, irritability, SIB.	Limited effectiveness.
Haloperidol	DA	Aggression, hyperactivity, impulsivity social relatedness, transitions, irritability/temper tantrums.	Risk for movement disorders (acute and chronic).
Risperidone	5-HT, DA	Aggression, hyperactivity/impulsivity, social relatedness, transitions, mood, irritability, temper tantrums, repetitive behaviors.	Weight gain, dose related drowsiness.

and friends, know intuitively that there is something wrong prior to the official diagnosis.

When parents are in different phases of the grieving process, communication between them becomes difficult. This may occur where one parent is still at a stage of denial and disbelief whilst the diagnosis has been accepted by the other parent, who is then trying to cope with a sense of loss and hopelessness.

At the time of diagnostic crisis there is need for a high level of social support to the family. If this is not available within the family social network, professional social work intervention is of paramount importance.

School Entry

School entry brings a set of challenges for parents with a child with PDD. Families who have been fortunate enough to participate in intensive early intervention programs, may have difficulty accessing a similar level of intervention in a school system. With most children being mainstreamed in regular classrooms parents and professionals must advocate for sufficient special education resources to meet the child's needs. Particularly in the early school years, intensive programming often requiring 1 :1 intervention, and computer assisted learning can be essential.

The **early school years** are often confusing for parents with an Asperger's Disorder child. The diagnosis may not be clear until the middle childhood years. Educators may interpret the child's social awkwardness, particularly their naïve tactless comments, as bad behavior. A diagnosis of Asperger's Disorder and appropriate advocacy by a well-trained professional is key to successful programming for these children.

Adolescence

Adolescence is a difficult time for the person with PDD and for their family. Hormonal changes with arousal of sexual and aggressive impulses and the management of menstruation and masturbation can be challenging. For lower functioning PDD individuals there is a wider gap between the comprehension and management of these novel urges and hormonal functions.

For higher functioning adolescents there is often an attempt to fit in with peers and there may be poor management of impulses. The intrinsic difficulty with social skills associated with these disorders complicates the tasks of adolescence and may result in feelings of hopelessness and even suicidal thoughts among teens with Asperger's Disorder. Inappropriate sexual expression such as inappropriate touching may create further difficulties for these youth. Academically the increased demand for abstract conceptualization accentuates the different learning needs of individuals with Asperger's Disorder and other high functioning PDD individuals.

Special education approaches in the high school curriculum continue to be an essential component of the habilitative process for low, medium and high functioning individuals with PDD. Functional academics, i.e., language, reading and math skills that enhance everyday function, along with the management of daily living routines are most likely to achieve the highest possible level of adult independence.

Transition to Adulthood

Successful **transition to adulthood** is best achieved through planning and programming during the adolescent years. Issues of placement, capacity for independent living, vocational opportunities and continued support services often absorb parental time and energy. The gap between intellectual ability and adaptive daily living skills particularly in the social area may mean that a high functioning individual becomes more comfortable in a vocational activity that may appear below his/her intellectual capability. With major curriculum adjustments and academic supports, a very high functioning PDD person may be able to enter a post secondary environment but this is the exception rather than the rule. Most important is to find contentment and a "niche" within adult society.

Summary

This chapter has reviewed the diagnostic features of autistic disorder and the other related PDDs. Issues of learning, communication, and vocational training have been explored. We have examined the vulnerabilities of these individuals and their effects on other family members. Discussion of day-to-day issues and the stresses of developmental transitions from childhood to adulthood provide an understanding of the life span trajectory for these individuals and their caregivers.

Resource Section

General Resource Texts

Handbook of Autism and Pervasive Developmental Disorders (2nd Edition). Edited by Donald J. Cohen and Fred R. Volkmar. John Wiley & Sons Inc., 1997.

Autism and Pervasive Developmental Disorders. Edited by Fred R. Volkmar. Cambridge University Press, 1998.

These texts are particularly useful for physicians and other professionals who are working with the PDD population.

Reading Resources List for Parents

Keys to Parenting the Child with Autism by Marlene Targ Brill. New York: Barron's Parenting Keys, 2nd Edition, 2001.
This book explains what autism/PDD is and how it is diagnosed. It provides advice on identifying resources, working with the therapeutic community, ensuring an appropriate education and helping each child with autism develop to his or her potential.

A Parent's Guide to Autism – Answers to the Most Common Questions by Charles A. Hart. New York: Pocket Books, Simon and Schuster Inc., 100 Front St., Riverside, NJ.
This book is presented in a question and answer format addressing symptoms and types of autism/PDD, possible causes, therapy options and treatment alternatives.

Children with Autism: A Parent's Guide by Michael D. Powers, MD. Kensington, MD: Woodbine House, 1989.
An informative and helpful guide for parents; Powers includes chapters on the diagnosis and treatment of Autism/PDD; adjusting to life with an autistic child; finding a good educational program; legal rights; becoming an advocate; and the adult with autism.

Asperger Syndrome & Your Child: A Parent's Guide by Michael D. Powers. New York: Harper Collins 2002.
Illustrated with engaging vignettes about children with Asperger Syndrome, this practical book has detailed advice for parents about supporting their young person's development.

Crossing Bridges: A Parent's Perspective on Coping After a child Is Diagnosed with Autism/PDD by Sarkiewicz-Gayherdt and others. Potential Unlimited Publishing Foundation, 1997.
This booklet, written by mothers of children with Autism/PDD, gives basic information about Autism/PDD and gives advice about how to access further information and support.

Navigating the Special Education System in Ontario: A Handbook for Parents of Children with Autism/PDD. Toronto: Autism Society Canada, 1996.
This handbook answers many questions that parents have regarding their child's education. The information is comprehensive and presented in a practical and user- friendly way.

Parents Survival Manual by Eric Schopler, New York: Plenum Press, 1995.
This book illustrates effective solutions to various behavior problems such as aggression, communication, perseveration, play, eating, sleeping, and hygiene.

Reading Resources for Families and Children

Siblings of Children with Autism: A Guide for Families by Sandra Harris, MD. Bethesda, MD: Woodbine House, 1994.
A useful book including chapters on brothers and sisters getting along, explaining autism to children, helping children share their feelings, finding time for family, work and yourself and helping children play together.

Russell is Extra Special by Charles A. Amenta. New York: Magination Press, 1992.
A wonderful book for young children and families. This book deals sensitively with the issue of an "invisible" handicap.

Please Don't Say Hello by Phyllis Gold. New York: Human Sciences Press, 1976.
This story depicts a family with two boys, one of whom is autistic, moving into a new neighborhood. The neighborhood children can see that Eddy is like them in many ways: he loves ice cream, playing basketball and splashing in the pool, but Eddy does some weird things that are hard to understand. The stress of telling new-found friends about one sibling and coping with their reactions is a major part of the story.

Joey and Sam by Illana Katz and Edward Ritvo. California Real Life Storybooks, 1993.
A heartwarming story about autism, a family and a brother's love.

Ian's Walk: A Story About Autism by Laurie Lears. Albert Whitman and Company, 1998.
A young girl's story about taking her brother (who has autism) for a walk to the park.

Inside Out by Ann M. Martin. New York: Scholastic Books, 1984.
Jonno's little brother is autistic. Lately, it seems that everything is getting spoiled because of James. Jonno just wants his life to be normal; he is tired of being laughed at by the "in kids." It isn't easy having a brother like James. Jonno hopes his life will change when James goes to a school for autistic children.

Captain Tommy by Abby Ward Messner. Potential Unlimited Publishing Foundation, 1996.
This book is about a young boy at summer camp who befriends a peer with autism.

Mixed Blessing by William and Barbara Christopher. Nashville, TN: Abingdon Press, 1989.
Two parents share the unforgettable story of their life raising two sons, John and Ned, and coming to the realization that Ned was not developing normally, eventually being diagnosed with autism.

Rainman by Leonore Fleischer. New York: Penguin Books Ltd., 1989.
Adapted for the screenplay "Rain Man," this is the story of Charles Babbitt who learns that his father left a legacy of three million dollars to an institutionalized brother he never knew. Charles kidnaps this brother, Raymond, in an attempt to get the money. The journey takes the pair back into the past, into loss and into an unexpected rebirth of love.

Laughing and Loving with Autism by Wayne Gilpin. Arlington, TX: Future Education Incorporated, 1993.
This book contains selections of humorous anecdotes written by parents of autistic children.

Without Reason by Charles Hart. New York: Harper and Row, 1989.
A story of a family coping with two generations of autism. The author demonstrates that it is possible to survive and even be strengthened after hearing the diagnosis of autism. He describes the lives of his brother and son with accuracy and empathy.

Simple Simon by Ann Lovell. Glasgow: Lyons Publishing, 1983.
A touching mother's story of a family, with an autistic member, told simply and without pretence.

Let Me hear Your Voice by Catherine Maurice. New York: Fawcett Columbia, 1994.
A beautifully written story by a mother of two autistic children, her efforts to help them and how they triumphed.

Reading Resources for Professionals and Parents

AspergerSyndrome: A Guide for Parents and Professionals by Tony Attwood. London: Jessica Kingsley Publishers, 1998.
This guide brings together the most relevant and useful information on all aspects of the syndrome, from language and social behavior to motor clumsiness with many examples of quotations from people with Asperger Syndrome.

High Functioning Individuals with Autism: Advice and Information for Parents and Others Who Care by Susan J. Moreno. Crown Point, IN: MAAP Services, 1991.
In this booklet, Moreno uses standard diagnostic criteria to describe the high functioning person with autism/PDD and then offers information and suggestions for issues at home, school and in the community.

The World of the Autistic Child by Bryna Siegal. New York: Oxford University Press, 1996.
This book thoroughly discusses a wide range of topics from diagnostic information to methods of treatment including medications. It is designed for parents and professionals.

Targeting Autism by Shirley Cohen. Berkeley: University of California Press, 1998.
This book discusses recent advances in early identification and educational treatment for children with autism. Ms. Cohen, an educator, looks at the many different approaches presently available, the current research findings and her own personal observations, as well as anecdotes from parents. The book is both realistic and hopeful.

The Importance of Early Diagnosis published by Autism Society Ontario, 1993.
This booklet defines autism and pervasive developmental disorder, describing what "autism looks like" and points to specific symptoms for children from newborn to 18 months, 1-1/2 to 4 years, and 4 years or older. The importance of early diagnosis and intervention are outlined.

Why Does Chris Do That? By Tony Attwood. London: The National Autistic Society, 1993.
Some suggestions regarding the cause and management of the unusual behavior of children and adults with autism and Asperger Syndrome.

Helpful Responses to Some of the Behaviors of Individuals with Autism by Nancy Darymple. Indiana University Press, 1992.
Presents many of the frequently encountered behavioral challenges associated with autism, together with an autism-specific interpretation of the behaviors and some potentially helpful responses.

Avoiding Unfortunate Situations by Dennis Debbaudt. Detroit: Autism Society of America, 1994.
A collection of experiences, tips and information from and about people with autism and other developmental disabilities and their encounters with law enforcement agencies.

Teaching Resources

Teaching Children with Autism by Kathleen Ann Quill. New York: Delmar Publishing Inc., 1995.
This book examines the learning styles of children with autism and offers a variety of teaching options with an emphasis on communication.

Teach Me Language by S. Freeman and L. Dake. SKF Books, 1996.
A language manual for children with PDD.

High Functioning Adolescents and Young Adults with Autism: A Teacher's Guide by Ann Fullarton et al. 8700 Shoal Creek Blvd., Austin, Texas 78757, Pro-Ed, 1996.
Included are chapters on defining and describing persons with Higher Functioning Autism, the impact of adolescent, strategies for assessing needs, organization and time management, and social assistance strategies.

Taming the Recess Jungle by Carol Gray. Michigan: Jenison Public Schools, 1993.
This book provides suggestions for socially simplifying recess for students with autism and related disorders.

Visual Strategies for Improving Communications. Volume 1. Practical Supports for School and Home. Quirk Robarts Publishing, P. O. Box 71, Troy, Michigan 48099-0071, 1995.
Describes numerous strategies to enhance communication interactions for students who experience autism and other moderate to severe communication disorders. This book describes specific strategies that capitalize on visual strengths and learning style of this population. Suitable for professionals and parents.

The Social Story Book. Michigan: Jenison Public Schools, 1994.
Social Stories are helpful in introducing new routines, explaining reasons for others' behavior and teaching social skills. This book has several stories, including personal care, cooking and meal-time routines, all about schools, restaurants and shopping, etc. Guidelines for writing, presenting and monitoring a social story are included.

Teaching Developmentally Disabled Children: The Me Book by Ivar O. Lovaas. Library of Congress Cataloguing in Publication Data: Pro-Ed, 8700 Shoal Creek Boulevard, Texas 78757.
This book is intended for parents and teachers. Should be helpful for persons with behavioral disabilities, be it as a result of a number of disorders (i.e., autism, emotional). Most programs were developed for children and youths. The early programs are laid out in considerable step-by-step detail.

Behavioral Interventions for Young Children with Autism. A Manual for Parents and Professionals Pro-Ed, Austin, Texas, 1996.

Included is choosing an effective treatment, what to teach, how to teach, who should teach, practical support re organizing and finding, working with a speech pathologist and working with schools.

Autism and Life in the Community: Successful Interventions for Behavioral Challenges. Baltimore: PH Brokes, 1990.
Issues in autism relating to behavioral assessment/intervention/modification, vocational skills, self-management, interpersonal skills and support services for community living are discussed.

Videotape Resources

Autism: A World Apart (VHS, 40 minutes, 1989)
Three families reflect on their older children with Autism. Issues of community placement and its ramifications are identified.

Portrait of an Autistic Young Man (VHS, 47 minutes, 1986) Produced by the Behavioral Sciences Media Laboratory, University of California.
Joseph Sullivan is a 24 year old who is unaware that he is autistic. He is the subject of this in-depth documentary study. The tape captures the peculiar symptomatology and lifestyle of a relatively functional yet severely disabled person. Portrait also records the struggles and accomplishments of Joseph's parents.

Autism – Little Victories (VHS, 28 minutes, 1992) Autism Society of British Columbia.
Autism is described and discussed by both parents and professionals.

Great Expectations – Living with more able Levels of Pervasive Developmental Disorder, (VHS, 35 minutes, 1996); Geneva Centre, Toronto, ON
Temple Grandin talks about her own experiences as a person with autism and gives advice for those working with individuals with high functioning Autism and Asperger Syndrome.

Education of Ashleigh Davies: Education and Integration (VHS, 17 minutes, 1992)
Autism British Columbia
A 12 year old autistic girl is integrated with her own individual education program.

Transitions: The Challenge of Change for Persons with Autism. (VHS, 15 minutes, 1992) Autism British Columbia
Examples and strategies for dealing with transitions are discussed. Several children with autism and their families are shown copies of specific transitions.

Lynn: a Little Girl goes to School (VHS, 29 minutes, 1982). Manitoba Department of Education.
This video follows Lynn, an autistic child integrated into a regular classroom, over a period of 18 months. Educational programming is discussed.

Good Work (VHS, 24 minutes, 1995) Autism Society of British Columbia
The benefits of using behavior therapy one discussed by parents and professionals. Early and consistent intervention are emphasized.

Brothers and Sisters (VHS, 21 minutes, 1995). Autism Society of British Columbia
A sibling of a child with autism narrates this video. Several siblings of varying ages discuss the rewards and challenges of living with autism.

Internet Resources

Centre for the Study of Autism
www.autism.com

Autism Society of Ontario
www.autismsociety.on.ca

Geneva Centre for Autism
www.autism.net
Kerry's Place Autism Services, Aurora, Ontario
k.p.autismservices@ci.on.ca

References

American Psychiatric Association (APA) (1980). *Diagnostic and statistical manual of mental disorders, 3rd edition.* Washington, DC: Author.

American Psychiatric Association (APA) (1994). *Diagnostic and statistical manual of mental disorders, 4th edition.* Washington, DC: Author.

American Psychiatric Association (APA) (1987). *Diagnostic and statistical manual of mental disorders, 3rd edition revised.* Washington, DC: Author.

Asperger, H. (1991). "Autistic psychopathy" in childhood. In U. Frith (Ed.), *Autism and Asperger syndrome* (pp.37-92). Translated and annotated by U. Frith. Cambridge: Cambridge University Press.

Bailey, A., Le Couteur, A., Gottesman I., Bolton P., Simonoff E., Yuzda E., et al. (1995). Autism as a strongly genetic disorder: Evidence from a British twin study. *Psychological Medicine, 25,* 63-77.

Bailey, A., Luthert, P., Bolton, P., Le Couteur, A., Rutter, M., & Harding, B. (1993). Autism and megalencephaly. *Lancet, 341,* 1225-1226.

Bailey, A., Phillips, W., & Rutter, M. (1996). Autism: Toward an integration of clinical, genetic, neuropsychological, and neurobiological perspectives. *Journal of Child Psychology and Psychiatry, 37,* 89-126.

Baron-Cohen, S. (1989). The autistic child's theory of mind: A case of specific developmental delay. *Journal of Child Psychology and Psychiatry, 30,* 285-297.

Barthelemy, C., Bruneau, N., & Conet-Eymard, J. M. (1988). Urinary free and conjugated catecholamines and metabolites in autistic children. *Journal of Autism and Developmental Disorders, 18,* 583-591.

Bishop, D.V.M. (1989). Asperger's syndrome and semantic-pragmatic disorder: Where are the boundaries? *British Journal of Communication, 24,* 107-121.

Bolton, P., Macdonald, H., Pickles, A., Rios P., Goode, S., Crowson, M., et al. (1994) A case-control family history study of autism. *Journal of Child Psychology & Psychiatry, 35,* 877-900.

Brook, S. I., & Bowler, D. M. (1992). Autism by another name? Semantic and pragmatic impairments in children. *Journal of Autism and Developmental Disorders, 22,* 61-81.

Cantor, D. S., Thatcher, R. W., Hrybyk, M.,& Kaye, H. (1986). Computerized EEG analyses of autistic children. *Journal of Autism and Developmental Disorders, 16,* 169-187.

Cantwell, D., Rutter, M., & Baker, L. (1978). Family factors. In M. Rutter and E. Schopler (Eds), *Autism: A reappraisal of concepts and treatment* (pp.269-296). New York: Plenum.

Carr, E. G., & Kemp, D. C. (1989). Functional equivalence of autistic leading and communicative, pointing: Analysis and treatment. *Journal of Autism and Developmental Disorders, 19,* 561-578.

Creak, M. (1963). Schizophrenic syndrome in childhood: Further progress of a working party. *Developmental Medical Child Neurology, 6,* 530-535.

De Long, G. R., & Dwyer, J. T. (1988). Correlation of family history with specific autistic subgroups: Asperger syndrome and bipolar affective disease. *Journal of Autism and Developmental Disorders, 18,* 593-600.

Ellis, H. D., Ellis, D. M., Fraser, W., & Deb, S. (1994). A preliminary study of right hemisphere cognitive deficits and impaired social judgments among young people with Asperger syndrome. *European Child and Adolescent Psychiatry, 3,* 255-266.

Fisman, S. N., Wolf, L. C., Ellison, D., & Freeman, T. (2000). A longitudinal study of siblings of children with chronic disabilities. *Canadian Journal of Psychiatry, 45,* 369-375.

Fisman, S. N., Wolf, L. C., Ellison, D., Gillis, B., Freeman, T., & Szatmari, P. (1996). Risk and protective factors affecting the adjustment of siblings of children with chronic disabilities. *Journal of American Academy of Child and Adolescent Psychiatry, 35,* 1532-1541.

Fisman, S. N., Wolf, L. C., & Noh, S. (1989). Marital intimacy in parents of exceptional children. *Canadian Journal of Psychiatry, 34,* 519-525.

Folstein, S., & Rutter, N. (1977). Infantile autism: A genetic study of 21 twin pairs. *Journal of Child Psychology and Psychiatry, 18,* 297-321.

Frith, U. (Ed). (1991). *Autism and Asperger Syndrome.* Cambridge UK: Cambridge University Press.

Gillberg, C. (1991). Outcome in autism and autistic-like conditions *Journal of American Academy of Child and Adolescent Psychiatry, 30,* 375-381.

Gillberg, C., Bjure, J., Uvebrant, P., & Vestergren, E. (1993). SPECT (Single Photon Emission Tomography) in 31 children and adolescents with autism and autistic-like conditions. *European Child and Adolescent Psychiatry, 2,* 50-59.

Gillberg, C., & Svennerholm, L. (1987). CSF monoamines in autistic syndromes and other pervasive developmental disorders of early childhood. *British Journal of Psychiatry, 151,* 89-94.

Green, J. (1990). Is Asperger's a syndrome? *Developmental Medicine and Child Neurology, 32,* 743-747.

Hameury, L., Roux, S., Barthelemy, C., Adrien, J. L., Desombre, H., Sauvage, D., et al. (1995) Quantified multidimensional assessment of autism and other pervasive developmental disorders. Application for bioclinical research. *European Child and Adolescent Psychiatry, 4,* 123-135.

Harris, S. L., & Handleman, J. S. (Eds). (1994). *Preschool education programs for children with autism.* Austin, TX: Pro-ED.

Jones, M. B., & Szatmari, P. (1988). Stoppage rules and genetic studies of autism. *Journal of Autism and Developmental Disorders, 20,* 241-248.

Kamps, D. M., Barbetta, P. M., Leonard, B. R., & Delquadri, J. (1994). Classwide peer tutoring: an integration strategy to improve reading skills and promote peer interaction among students with autism and general education peers. *Journal of Applied Behavior Analysis, 27,* 49-61.

Kanner, L. (1943). Autistic disturbances of affective contact. *Nervous Child, 2,* 217-250.

Koegel, L. K., Koegel, R. L., Hurley, C., & Frea, W.D. (1992). Improving social skills and disruptive behavior in children with autism through self-management. *Journal of Applied Behavior Analysis, 25,* 341-353.

Kolvin, I. (1971). Studies in the childhood psychosis. Diagnostic criteria and classification. *British Journal of Psychiatry, 118,* 381-384.

Leiter, R. G. (1948) *Leiter international performance scale.* Chicago, IL: Stoelting.

Leventhal, B. L., Cook, E. H. Jr., Morford, M., Ravitz, A., & Freedman, D. X. (1990). Relationships of whole blood serotonin and plasma norepinephrine within families. *Journal of Autism and Developmental Disorders, 20,* 499-511.

Lord, C., & Rutter, M. (1994). Autism and pervasive developmental disorders. In M. Rutter, E. Taylor & L. Herson (Eds), *Child and adolescent psychiatry, modern approaches* (pp.569-593). London, UK: Blackwell.

Lord, C., Rutter, M., Goode, S., Heemsberger, J., Jordan, H., Mawhood, L , et al. (1989). Autism diagnostic observation schedule: a standardized observation of communicative and social behavior. *Journal of Autism and Developmental Disorders, 19,* 185-212.

Lord, C., Rutter, M., & Le Couteur, A. (1994). Autism Diagnostic Interview-revised. A revised version of a diagnostic interview for caregivers of individuals with possible pervasive developmental disorders. *Journal of Autism and Developmental Disorders, 24,* 659-685.

Lovaas, O. I. (1987). Behavioral treatment and normal educational and intellectual functioning in young autistic children. *Journal of Consulting and Clinical Psychology, 55,* 3-9.

Martineau, J., Barthelemy, C., Jouve, J., Muh, J. P., & Lelord, G. (1992). Monoamines (serotonin and catecholamines) and their derivatives in infantile autism: Age-related changes and drug effects. *Developmental Medical Child Neurology, 34,* 595-603.

Mason, S. S., McGee, G. G., Farmer-Dougan, V., & Risley, T.,R. (1989). A practical strategy for ongoing reinforcer assessment. *Jouranl of Applied Behavior Analysis, 22,* 171-179.

Noh, S., Dumas, J. E., Wolf, L. D., & Fisman, S. N. (1989). Delineating sources of stress in parents of exceptional children. *Family Relations, 38,* 456-461.

Ozonoff, S., & McEvoy, E. E. (1994). A longitudinal study of executive dysfunction and theory of mind development in autism. *Development and Psychopathology, 6,* 415-431.

Panksepp, J., & Sahley, T. L. (1987). Possible brain opiod involvement in disrupted social intent and language development in autism. In E. Schopler & G. B. Mesibov (Eds), *Neurobiological issues in autism* (pp. 357-372). New York, NY: Plenum Press.

Pickles, A., Bolton, P., Macdonald, H., Bailey, A., Le Couteur A, Sim, C. H., et al. (1995). Latent-class analysis of recurrence risks for complex phenotypes with selection and measurement error: A twin and family history study of autism. *American Journal of Medical Genetics, 57,* 717-726.

Pierce, K., & Shreibman, L. (1994). Teaching daily living skills to children with autism in unsupervised settings through pictorial self-management. *Journal of Applied Behavior Analysis, 27,* 471-481.

Piven, J., Arndt, S., Bailey, J., & Andreasen, N. (1996). Regional brain enlargement in autism: A magnetic resonance imaging study. *Journal of American Academy of Child and Adolescent Psychiatry, 35,* 530-536.

Piven, J., Arndt, S., Bailey, J., Havercamp, S., Andreasen, N. C., & Palmer, P. (1995). An MRI study of brain size in autism. *American Journal of Psychiatry, 152,* 1145-1149.

Piven, J., Saliba, K., Bailey, J. & Arndt, S. (1997). An MRI study of autism: The cerebellum revisited. *Neurology, 49,* 546-551.

Piven, J., Wzorek, M., Landa, R., Lainhart, J., Bolton, P., Chase, G.A., et al. (1994). Personality characteristics of the parents of autistic individuals. *Psychological Medicine, 24,* 783-795.

Ritvo, E. R., Spence, M. A., Freeman, B. J., Mason-Brothers, A., Mo, A., & Marazita, M. I. (1985). Evidence for autosomal recessive inheritance in 46 families with multiple incidences of autism. *American Journal of Psychiatry, 142,* 187-192.

Rourke, B. (1989). *Nonverbal learning disabilities: The syndrome and the model.* New York, NY: Guilford Press.

Rutter, M., & Schopler, E. (1992). Classification of pervasive developmental disorders: Some concepts of practical consideration. *Journal of Autism and Developmental Disorders, 22,* 459-482.

Schuler, A. L., Prizant, B. M., & Wetherby, A. M. (1997). Enhancing language and communication development: Prelinguistic approaches. In D. Cohen & F. Volkmar (Eds), *Handbook of autism and pervasive developmental disorders* (2nd ed.). (pp. 539-571). New York, NY: John Wiley & Sons, Inc.

Semrud-Clikeman, M., & Hynd, G. W. (1990). Right hemispheric dysfunction in nonverbal learning disabilities: Social, academic, and adaptive functioning in adults and children. *Psychological Bulletin, 197,* 196-209.

Short, A. B., & Schopler, E. (1988). Factors relating to age of onset in autism. *Journal of Autism and Developmental Disorders, 18,* 207-216.

Sigman, M., Arbelle, S., & Dissanayake, C. (1995). Current research findings in childhood autism. *The Canadian Journal of Psychiatry, 40,* 289-294.

Smalley, S. L., Asarnow, R. F., & Spence, M. A. (1988). Autism and genetics: A decade of research. *Archives of General Psychiatry, 45,* 953-961.

Smalley, S. L., McCracken, J., & Tanguay, P. (1995). Autism, affective disorders, and social phobia. *American Journal of Medical Genetics, 60,* 19-26.

Sparrow, S. S., Balla, D. & Cicchetti, D. V. (1984). *Vineland Adaptive Behavior Scales* (expanded form). Circle Pines, MN: American Guidance Service.

Steffenburg, S., Gillberg, C., Hellgren, L., Andersson, L., Gillberg, I. C., Jakobsson, G., et al. (1989). A twin study of autism in Denmark, Finland, Iceland, Norway, and Sweden. *Journal of Child Psychology and Psychiatry, 30,* 405-416.

Stowitscheck, J. J. (1992). Policy and planning in transition programs at the state agency level. In F.R. Rusch, L. DeStefano, L. Chadsey-Rusch, A. Phelps, & E. Syzmanski (Eds), *Transition from school to adult life: Models, linkages, and policy* (pp. 519-536). Sycamore, IL: Sycamore.

Szatmari, P., Archer, L., Fisman, S., Streiner, D. L., & Wilson, F. (1995). Asperger syndrome and autism: Differences in behavior, cognition, and adaptive functioning. *Journal of American Academy of Child and Adolescent Psychiatry, 34,* 1662-1671.

Szatmari, P., Jones, M. B., Fisman, S., Tuff, L., Bartolucci, G., Mahoney, W. J., et al. (1995). Parents and collateral relatives of children with pervasive developmental disorders: A family history study. *American Journal of Medical Genetics, 60,* 282-289.

Szatmari, P., Jones, M. B., Tuff, L., Bartolucci, G., Fisman, S., & Mahoney W. (1993). Lack of cognitive impairment in first-degree relatives of children with pervasive developmental disorders. *Journal of American Academy of Child and Adolescent Psychiatry, 32,* 1264-1273.

Szelazek, J. T., Williamson, P. C., Fisman, S., Steele, M., Gati, J. S., Densmore, R. S., et al. (2000). Regional brain functioning during verbal fluency tasks in subjects with Asperger's Disorder. Published abstract in conference proceedings *Beyond 2000: Healthy tomorrows for children and youth.* Ottawa, ON.

Tantum, D. (1991). Asperger syndrome in adulthood. In U. Frith (ed.), *Autism and Asperger syndrome* (pp. 147-183). Cambridge, UK: Cambridge University Press.

Ventner, A., Lord, C., & Schopler, E. (1992). A follow-up of high functioning autistic children. *Journal of Child Psychology and Psychiatry, 33,* 489-507.

Volkmar, F. R., Cicchetti, D. V., Bregman, J., & Cohen, D. J. (1992). Three diagnostic systems for autism: DSM-III, DSM-IV, and ICD-10. *Journal of Autism and Developmental Disorders, 22,* 483-492.

Waterhouse, L., & Fein, D. (1997). Perspectives on social impairment. In D. Cohen & F. R. Volkmar (Eds.), *Developmental disorders: A handbook* (pp. 909-1019). New York, NY: John Wiley.

Wing, L. (1981). Asperger's syndrome. A clinical account. *Psychological Medicine, 11,* 115-129.

Wing, L. (1986). Letter: Clarification of Asperger's syndrome. *Journal of Autism and Developmental Disorders, 16,* 513-515.

Wing, L., & Gould, J. (1979). Severe impairments of social interaction and associated abnormalities in children. Epidemiology and classification. *Journal of Autism and Developmental Disorders, 9,* 11-29.

Wolf, L. C., Fisman, S. N., & Ellison, D. (1998). Effect of differential parental treatment in sibling dyads with one disabled child: A longitudinal perspective. *Journal of American Academy of Child and Adolescent Psychiatry, 37,* 1317-1325.

Wolf, L. C., Noh, S., Fisman, S. N., & Speechley, M. (1989). Psychological effects of parenting stress on parents of autistic children. *Journal of Autism and Developmental Disorders, 19,* 157-166.

World Health Organization (WHO) (1990). Criteria for Research (draft). In *International classification of diseases, 10th edition (ICD-10): Classification of mental and behavioral disorders.* Geneva, SW: Author.

Zibovicius, M., Garreau, B., Samson, Y., Remy, P., Barthelemy, C., Syrota, A., et al. (1995). Delayed maturation of the frontal cortex in childhood autism. *American Journal of Psychiatry, 152,* 248-252.

CHAPTER 7

22q Deletion Syndrome

Kerry Boyd, Anne Bassett, Lonnie Zwaigenbaum, & Eva Chow

Introduction

22q11.2 Deletion Syndrome (22qDS), as the name implies, is a genetic disorder involving a small missing piece (deletion) from Chromosome 22. This can result in multiple congenital anomalies (birth defects) and developmental challenges with substantial variability among individuals with 22qDS. This syndrome is relatively common, particularly among those dually diagnosed with developmental disability and mental health disorders. Even with recent advances in genetic testing and clinical recognition, there are many individuals who carry this genetic deletion who remain undiagnosed as adults. Given the prevalence, wide-ranging manifestations and lifelong disability associated with 22qDS, increased knowledge regarding early identification and on-going management will be important to health care providers, mental health professionals, educators and other members of multidisciplinary teams.

Timely recognition of 22qDS can aid identification of a number of important and under-recognized medical conditions, guide assessment and remediation of cognitive deficits as well as alert caregivers and mental health professionals to psychiatric and medical vulnerabilities associated with this syndrome.

This chapter will outline the history of the syndrome's delineation, the genetic etiology, the clinical features including the potential for multi-system involvement, developmental and neurocognitive profiles, and the psychiatric issues which a portion of affected individuals face.

Historical Overview

To appreciate the significance of the discovery of the microdeletion on Chromosome 22 it is useful to look at the history of the syndrome's delineation before and after that discovery.

Dr. Eva Sedlackova reported a series of patients with soft palate, facial and, sometimes, cardiac anomalies in a Czech language journal in 1955. In 1968 Dr. William Strong described four members of one family with cardiac anomalies, learning disabilities and noteworthy facial features. Other isolated case reports and case series describing individuals with similar characteristics can be found in journals in the 1970's and 1980's.

DiGeorge Syndrome (DGS) was named after paediatric endocrinologist Dr. Angelo DiGeorge. In the 1960's he described a constellation of findings in infants he saw with low serum calcium levels and recurrent infections secondary to problems with the thymus gland. A proportion had congenital heart defects and could manifest palatal anomalies. Another name was given to the syndrome in 1976 by Dr. Kinouchi in Japan, who described patients with a category of heart defects known as conotruncal anomalies in association with some consistent facial features. He called this **Conotruncal Anomaly Face Syndrome (CTAFS)**.

In 1978, Robert Shprintzen, Ph.D., a speech pathologist, described a series of patients with cleft palate or velopharyngeal incompetence, congenital cardiac defects, some similar facial characteristics and learning disabilities. He gave a descriptive title of **Velocardiofacial Syndrome (VCFS)**, though it has since also been referred to as **Shprintzen Syndrome**. Geneticist, Dr. Tony Lipson, described a number of patients with VCFS, noting variability of features among those with the syndrome, even within affected families. During the 1980's and early 1990's there were again and again reports in the literature by a number of clinicians observing the overlap among descriptions of DGS, CTAFS and VCFS. Further, ear, nose and throat specialists had added **Opitz G/BBB Syndrome** to the list with apparent similarities in features.

Genetic discoveries in the early 1980's began the process of clarifying the underlying cause (Lindsay et al., 1995; Scambler et al., 1992). In 1981 Dr. de la Chapelle in France and in 1982 Drs. Richard Kelley, Elaine Zackai and Beverly Emanuel from the Children's Hospital of Philadelphia (C.H.O.P.) looked at selected DGS cases and found in some a visible deletion on chromosome 22 when examined under a microscope. Dr. Emanuel's team followed up on this discovery and found that 25% of patients with DGS had this visible chromosome 22 deletion but 75% did not. It was not until 1991 that Dr. Debra Driscoll and Dr. Emanuel's team discovered, using a more sensitive molecular test, that there actually was a deletion too small to be detectable by the microscope alone. A molecular DNA test called fluorescence in-situ hybridization (FISH) was used to verify the presence of this "microdeletion."

The discovery of the 22q deletion and the use of FISH to identify the microdeletion has helped to clarify many issues. In particular, those described as having CTAFS, VCFS, and DGS usually have the same deletion on chromosome 22 as the underlying cause for cardiac, other medical and physical features. The name given to the syndrome historically seemed to depend on the specialty or type of clinical service evaluating the person. Those who received clinical diagnoses of these syndromes are generally tested for the deletion. The collective acronym **CATCH 22** was initially suggested for those with a verified 22q deletion to emphasize the more prominent congenital features seen primarily in DGS (**C**ardiac anomalies, **A**bnormal facies, **T**hymic hypoplasia, **C**left palate and **H**ypocalcemia) (Hall, 1993; Wilson, Burn, Scambler, & Goodship, 1993). Case series have highlighted a much wider range of potential features involving other body systems (Lipson et al., 1991; Ravnan, Chen, Golabi, & Lebo, 1996; Shprintzen, Goldberg, Young, & Wolford, 1981). Among those ascertained in adulthood presenting with psychiatric symptoms, the physical features can be subtle (Bassett, Hodgkinson, Chow, Correia, Scutt & Weksberg, 1998). Therefore, it seems preferable to use **22q deletion Syndrome (22qDS)** to emphasize the underlying etiology and thus to allow researchers and clinicians to be referring to a uniform group of patients.

The Genetics of 22qDS

People with 22qDS have a normal number of chromosomes, ie. 23 pairs, one from each parent. The autosome pairs are numbered 1 through 22 and the 23rd pair are sex chromosomes determining, among other things, whether the person will be male or female.

The deletion of interest in this syndrome occurs on chromosome 22, the smallest of the autosomes. The specific region is referred to by geneticists as 22q11.2 which locates the deletion on the long arm ("q" arm) of chromosome 22 and at a specific region on band 11.2. A DNA probe designed to attach to this region is used in the fluorescence in-situ hybridization (FISH) test. The fluorescently labelled probe "seeks out" the q11.2 region on chromosome 22 and if it is missing (deleted) only the intact chromosome 22 will show this region under the fluorescent microscope (a positive FISH test for 22qDS).

Research is ongoing to isolate specific genes within the deleted region, to determine their function, the consequences of haploinsuffiency (loss of one gene copy) and how this may translate into the clinical features. There are over 30 genes in the 22q11.2 deletion region. Most of these have been characterized and several are known to have important functions during embryonic and fetal development, e.g., TBX1 (T-box 1, a transcription factor), and throughout life in brain functioning, e.g., COMT (catechol-O-methyltransferase) (Lindsay, 2001). However, it is not yet known which gene or combination of genes are responsible for the clinical features of 22qDS (Lindsay, 2001).

Figure 1. Fluorescence In-Situ Hybridization (FISH) for common deletions in 22q Deletion Syndrome (22qDS)

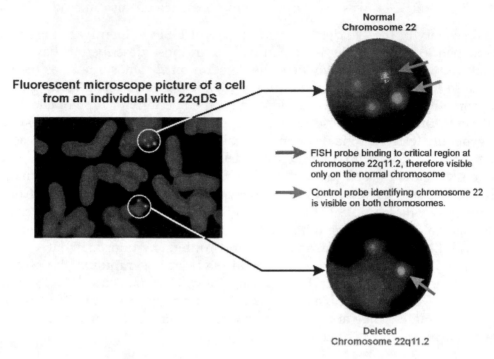

What remains poorly understood, and to be further studied, is why there is so much variability in the phenotype (physical and behavioural expression) and why the severity of features is unrelated to the size or exact position of the deletion. One way to study gene expression is using a mouse model which takes advantage of the fact that the gene content of the chromosome 22q11.2 region is similar in the mouse genome. This has allowed researchers to generate deletions in the mouse comparable to those in 22qDS. Mice with these deletions show certain birth defects, such as congenital cardiac defects, but other physical features of 22qDS are absent (Lindsay, 2001). Interestingly, like humans, only a proportion of mice with chromosomal deletions have visible cardiac defects (Lindsay, 2001). Mouse models may continue to shed light on the involvement of specific genes in phenotype expression. However these models have limited utility in the study of complex behavioural manifestations of 22qDS.

It also remains to be clarified why some individuals with the clinical features of the syndrome (eg. VCFS, DGS) have a negative FISH test for the 22q11.2 deletion using the standard clinical probe (eg. TUPLE1). Some atypical deletions in the 22q11.2 region are detectable on a research basis using other probes. There may be other deletion sites, more complex genetic mechanisms, interactions with, as yet, undetermined influences, or mosaicism (not all blood cells or tissues have the deletion). Also, non-deleted individuals who have the clinical features of 22qDS may have other conditions such as fetal alcohol syndrome (Demczuk & Aurias, 1995; Lindsay, 2001).

Transmission

Most (approximately 9 in 10) people identified with a 22q11.2 deletion are the first in their family to have this syndrome and did not inherit the deletion from a parent. Thus, in a majority of individuals the missing genetic material represents a "new (or de novo) mutation", i.e., it occurs spontaneously and is new to the family. It is not the result of anything that happened during pregnancy, labour/delivery or after birth, but rather is a change that occurred prior to conception during gametogenesis, i.e., in the formation of the mother's ovum (egg) or father's sperm. Although the exact cause of new deletions is currently unknown, researchers have identified "low copy repeat" segments of DNA on either side of the typically deleted segment which appear to make the region prone to genetic mutations (changes) or rearrangements (Edelmann et al., 1999). A similar mechanism may be responsible for deletions in Williams, Prader-Willi, Angelman and Smith Magenis syndromes (Lindsay, 2001).

Once an individual has been diagnosed with the deletion, families should meet with a genetic counsellor (Hodgkinson, Murphy, O'Neill, Brzustowicz, & Bassett, 2001). It is also recommended that the parents be tested genetically (Hodgkinson et al., 2001). In about 10% of individuals the deletion has been inherited from a parent. Parents with a deletion often have no obvious features of the syndrome and therefore may have been undetected (McDonald-McGinn et al., 2001). Transmission of a 22q11.2 deletion is in an autosomal dominant pattern; that is, an individual who carries the deletion has a 50% risk of passing it on with each conception (Hodgkinson et al., 2001). Fertility does not appear to be affected by 22qDS, although severely affected individuals may have decreased social opportunities to have partners. In all cases, the severity of expression of the missing genetic material is variable and cannot be predicted (Hodgkinson et al., 2001). See Table 1.

Table 1: The Genetics of 22qDS

- ♦ Most deletions arise *de novo* - cause unknown
- ♦ About 10% have been inherited from a parent
- ♦ Autosomal dominant pattern of inheritance - deletion transmitted to 50% of offspring
- ♦ Variable expression
- ♦ Research ongoing to understand underlying genetic mechanisms

How Common Is 22q Deletion Syndrome?

As noted above, several syndromes described in the literature are associated with 22q11.2 deletions. These include VCFS, DGS and CTAFS (Demczuk & Aurias, 1995; Driscoll et al., 1993; Kelly et al., 1993; Lindsay et al., 1995; Scambler et al., 1992). Prevalence has been estimated at 1/4,000 live births (Goodship, Cross, LiLing, & Wren, 1998), based on a newborn population with recognizable congenital heart defects, which is likely to be an underestimate given that many individuals with

22qDS have no heart defect. As such, 22qDS is likely the most common microdeletion syndrome currently known (Lindsay, 2001). Increasingly in the field there is an emphasis on the variability of presentations and the need to test families of affected individuals who may be carriers of the deletion and have no obvious features. C.H.O.P. describes a group of 30 individuals identified with the deletion because of an affected family member, many of whom had no major clinical clues that would have suggested a diagnosis of 22qDS. The authors suggest the prevalence of 22qDS may be much higher than previous estimates and recommended clinicians "cast a wide FISHing net" (McDonald-McGinn et al., 2001). Additionally, it would appear that 22q deletions are under-recognized among those with developmental delays and/or psychiatric problems, most notably psychotic disorders (Bassett & Chow, 1999; Bassett, Chow, & Weksberg, 2000). It has been observed that in this population the physical phenotype may be less recognizable at an early age and, therefore, would represent a subgroup so far not included in the prevalence estimates.

Clinical Features of 22qDS

This section will serve as an overview of the range of features observed in individuals with 22qDS. The work is ongoing, nonetheless there is a great deal of useful information to assist in identifying the syndrome and for supporting individuals already diagnosed.

It is important to note that there is considerable variability among those with 22qDS. The prevalence of various symptoms reported in the literature varies based on how the individuals were initially identified (e.g., due to palatal problems versus congenital heart defect). As well, ascertainment through hospital-based specialty clinics (i.e., palate, cardiac, endocrine, immunology) may select individuals with more severe medical problems. As noted earlier, people with 22qDS identified through an affected relative generally have a milder phenotype (Cohen, Chow, Weksberg, & Bassett, 1999; McDonald-McGinn et al., 2001). It is, therefore, difficult to give frequency estimates of the main features which would apply across all clinical settings. For example, rates of congenital heart defects have often been reported to be about 75-80% (Ryan et al., 1998), but in samples ascertained mainly through sources other than paediatric cardiac clinics this rate is 35-40% (Cohen et al., 1999).

Facial and Other Minor Physical Features

Facial features described in VCFS by Shprintzen et.al, (1981) include long face, narrow palpebral fissures (eye openings), broad nasal bridge, a prominent tubular nose with a bulbous nasal tip, a small, open mouth, and retrognathia (retruded chin). Small ears are also very common (Scutt, Chow, Weksberg, Honer, & Bassett, 2001), often with an overfold at the top. The facial features in 22qDS can be subtle, vary from person to person, and therefore take experience to recognize. The typical facial appearance tends to change with age. Slender hands with thin, tapered fingers are characteristic but not often present. See Table 2.

Table 2: Facial Features in 22qDS

- ◆ Narrow palpebral fissures
- ◆ Small ears (+/- minor ear anomalies)
- ◆ Prominent nose with bulbous tip
- ◆ Small mouth (often open posture)
- ◆ Small, retruded jaw
- ◆ Long face

Palate and Velopharyngeal Problems

There is a range of problems that can be associated with the palate. An overt cleft palate is easily detectable in infancy. However, it is increasingly recognized that more subtle problems are more often associated with 22qDS. A submucosal cleft palate is less readily identifiable because the mucous membrane of the mouth covers the separation of the palate. Most common in 22qDS is velopharyngeal incompetence (VPI) (velum referring to the soft palate and pharynx meaning throat) that involves incoordination of the muscles of the palate and throat, leading to hypernasal-sounding speech. These anomalies of the structure or functioning of the palate and pharynx can present in infancy as difficulties with sucking/feeding, regurgitation of food through the nose, or a hypernasal voice/cry, but often may not be recognized until school age. Speech therapy and in many cases specific surgery are often helpful. Other anomalies, including a bifid (split) uvula occur and have no functional significance but may suggest an underlying submucous cleft palate.

Gastrointestinal

Incoordination of musculature resulting in abnormal movement (dysmotility) can also be found in the esophagus. This, together with VPI, can further contribute to feeding problems and may be a risk factor for poor weight gain, particularly in the first year of life (Digilio, Marino, Cappa, Cambiaso, Giannotti & Dallapiccola, 2001). Vomiting and gagging may occur later on. Constipation is another frequent problem in 22qDS.

Researchers have observed dysmotility problems affecting various parts of the gastrointestinal tract. About 30% of children studied had feeding problems mainly in the first 3 years of life (Gerdes, Solot, Wang, McDonald-McGinn, & Zackai, 2001). X-ray studies revealed dysmotility of the throat and esophagus as well as gastroesophageal reflux and delayed gastric (stomach) emptying (Eicher et al., 2000). Over time, improvement was noted in some cases with specific treatments, for example for reflux, delayed gastric emptying or constipation.

Cardiac

Congenital cardiac (heart) defects are common in individuals with 22qDS (Goldmuntz et al., 1998). There is a range of severity with some aortic or septal defects going undetected. More major defects are usually noticed in the first year of life. Tetralogy of Fallot is particularly common. This is a complex of four congenital heart defects, ie. aorta is in a different position, the pulmonary artery has a stenosis (narrowing), the septum that divides the heart's ventricular chambers has a hole in it (ventricular septal defect), and the walls of the right ventricle are hypertrophied (thick). Other heart defects which are associated with 22qDS include isolated ventricular septal defect, abnormalities in the pulmonary artery, and complex transposition of the great arteries (the relationship between the ventricular chambers, and the aorta and pulmonary artery, is inverted with respect to the usual anatomy). Other abnormalities of the structure or location of the large blood vessels may be found (Boudjemline, Fermont, Le Bidois, Lyonnet, Side, & Bonnet, 2001). Most defects are now surgically correctable, although rarely some may be lethal in the neonatal period.

Immunology

Individuals with 22qDS may also have significant deficiencies involving the immune system, due to decreased growth or absence of the thymus gland prior to birth (Sullivan, 2001). Historically most children with this clinical profile have been diagnosed with DiGeorge Syndrome. The thymus gland produces T-cells, an important type of white blood cells (WBC) that are needed to fight infections and to mount an immune response to vaccinations. While severe immunodeficiency is rare in 22qDS, milder problems with the immune system are relatively common in childhood (e.g., presenting as recurrent respiratory tract infections) (Sullivan, 2001). It is important to screen for these problems (Swillen, Vogels, Devriendt, & Fryns, 2000). Autoimmune disorders have also been reported, but long-term follow-up studies are needed to determine the frequency of such disorders as hypothyroidism, hyperthyroidism, idiopathic thrombocytopenia, celiac disease, inflammatory bowel disease and arthritis in 22qDS adults (Swillen et al., 2000).

Endocrine

Hypocalcemia (low blood calcium levels) may result from abnormalities in the development and functioning of the parathyroid gland. This gland produces parathyroid hormone that is important for maintaining calcium levels in the body. Hypocalcemia may be detected in infancy and may initially present with symptoms such as irritability or seizures. The low calcium levels should be diagnosed and treated through periodic evaluations by an endocrinologist. This problem can subside, but may recur. Low calcium may also be first detected during the adult years. It is therefore recommended that ionized calcium and parathyroid hormone levels should be regularly monitored in 22qDS (Bassett & Chow, 1999; Weinzimer, 2001). It may be particularly important to recheck calcium levels in times of stress (Goldberg, Motzkin, Marion, Scambler, & Shprintzen, 1993).

Other hormone deficiencies have also been noted in 22qDS. Hypothyroidism can occur, and more rarely hyperthyroidism has been reported (Weinzimer, 2001). These occur mainly as a result of abnormal production of antithyroid antibodies (autoimmune) rather than faulty development of the thyroid. They are likely to be more common in adulthood (Bassett et al., 1998), and regular monitoring of thyroid stimulating hormone (TSH) is recommended for those with 22qDS. Growth hormone deficiencies have been noted in a small minority of children with 22qDS (Weinzimer, 2001).

Case Study #1

David was born following an uncomplicated full-term pregnancy and delivery in the early 1990's. He was noted in the delivery room to have a right-sided cleft lip and palate, and soon afterwards was found to have a heart murmur that was subsequently diagnosed as a ventricular septal defect. His cleft lip was repaired when he was 4 months of age, and his palate, at 1 year. Around that time, he was noted to be delayed in his motor milestones, and was referred to the local infant development program. Psychometric assessment at 15 months of age indicated mild delays in language and motor skills. He was a cheerful and energetic infant who enjoyed social play, but his vocalization consisted primarily of vowel sounds, and he was not yet walking or picking up small objects. He continued to make steady progress during the preschool years, although continued to show significant delays in speech sound development and language skills. His general health was good, although he did have recurrent ear infections and some feeding difficulties, and was slow to gain weight.

David was initially seen by a clinical geneticist at 18 months of age. At that time he was noted to have distinctive facial features including protuberant ears with simplified helices (outer ear structure), broad nasal bridge, and a slightly flattened facial profile (see photograph taken at 4 years of age). The significance of the concurrence of cleft lip and palate, and his congenital heart defect was noted. Routine analysis of his chromosomes was reported to be normal (i.e., no deletion was observed under the microscope under standard resolution). He was reassessed at the age of 5 years, and noted to have persistent developmental delays, as well as difficulty keeping up to peers academically in his kindergarten class. His height and weight also continued to be near the lower end of the growth curves, despite average adult height of both parents. The diagnosis of 22q DS was confirmed by FISH testing. This test had not been commercially available when David was initially assessed by the geneticist. Further investigation including abdominal ultrasound and measurement of serum calcium and immune factors were all within normal limits.

Despite improvements in language skills, David's repertoire of speech sounds remained quite limited. The hypernasal quality of his voice also became increasingly apparent, contributing to David's difficulty making himself understood (i.e., poor intelligibility of his speech). Assessment of velo-pharyngeal function (ability to obtain a seal between the posterior palate and pharyngeal wall) was abnormal. There was inadequate velo-pharyngeal closure during speech, consistent with velopharyngeal insufficiency. Surgical intervention (grafting of additional tissue, or 'pharyngeal flap', to aid closure) at the age of 7 years helped reduce hypernasal tone of David's speech, and improve his verbal intelligibility. Prior to surgery, the location of David's carotid arteries (large blood vessels that extend from the aorta into the neck) was confirmed. Among the various blood vessel anomalies that may be observed in 22qDS is internal displacement of the carotid arteries towards the surface of the pharyngeal wall, making surgical intervention more risky.

David has continued to experience difficulties at school. He has required a modified academic program, although remains integrated into the regular stream with the support of an educational aide. Psychoeducational assessment at age 7 years indicated that David's overall intellectual abilities were at the 1st percentile. There was a significant discrepancy between various domains of ability, with verbal reasoning skills being more advanced than visual spatial reasoning. He has also exhibited significant difficulties with his concentration, organizational skills, and impulse control. He is very distractible, has difficulty waiting his turn, and needs reminders to follow basic safety rules (e.g., running out into the street to retrieve a ball). At the age of 8 years, he participated in a research study of social and emotional development of children with 22qDS. Formal assessment using standardized measures was consistent with a DSM-IV diagnosis of Attention Deficit Hyperactivity Disorder. He showed a positive response to stimulant medication following a double blind placebo controlled trial, and remained on a low dose of that medication with some improvement in attention and behaviour at school.

Brain Development/Neurological Symptoms

Seizures may be present in 22qDS and may or may not be related to hypocalcemia. Other neurological symptoms have been reported in association with this syndrome, but are rare. These include hemiparesis (weakness on one side) of facial muscles or limbs, myoclonus and tremors have also been reported (Bassett et al., 1998). Ataxia (unsteady gait) may be a late developing feature in adults (Chow et al., 1999).

Magnetic resonance imaging (MRI) studies have been used to assess whether individuals with 22qDS show differences in brain structure. These studies have found a wide range of anomalies such as cortical and cerebellar atrophy, enlarged ventricles, and increased rates of normal variants such as local bright foci and cavum vergae (Chow et al., 1999; Mitnick, Bello, & Shprintzen, 1994). There are also individual case reports of associations of 22qDS with various structural brain anomalies (Chow et al., 1999).

Studies are ongoing to attempt to localize structural brain changes that may be associated with the cognitive deficits and psychiatric illnesses of 22qDS. Changes during brain development must, however, be taken into account. For example, decreased white matter volume was prominent in one study involving children with 22qDS (Eliez et al., 2001). However, a study involving adults with 22qDS and schizophrenia found that gray matter volumes were significantly reduced, while white matter volumes were similar to those in healthy controls (Chow, Zipursky, Mikulis, & Bassett, 2002). Enlarged ventricles were also found to be associated with psychotic illness in 22qDS (Chow et al., 2002). Longitudinal studies of children with 22qDS are underway to separate normal developmental brain changes from those associated with psychiatric illness.

Other

22qDS has many other associated features, potentially involving any organ system and presenting at birth or later in life. Some of the more commonly associated features include decreased platelet counts, usually in the low normal range, but sometimes in the below normal (thromocytopenia) range, though only rarely associated with bleeding problems (Lazier et al., 2001). Abnormalities of the kidneys and/or urinary system are relatively common (about 20% to 35% of individuals with 22qDS). An ultrasound is recommended for anyone diagnosed with 22qDS. There are a variety of connective tissue or limb-related problems, including cervical spine and other vertebral anomalies, patellar dislocations, joint laxity or contractures, club foot, polydactyly, and varicose veins. Other common musculoskeletal system conditions include scoliosis (curvatures of the spine), found in about 10% of patients (Swillen et al., 2000). Hearing problems may be secondary to ear infections and/or involve congenital sensorineural hearing loss, thus assessment of hearing is important in 22qDS. With respect to growth abnormalities, slow weight gain, sometimes diagnosed as failure to thrive, may be observed in the first years of life due to feeding problems, associated medical conditions or possibly due to direct effects of the deletion on growth. This may be followed by a period of normal growth. Short stature is reported in 10% of children but normal height is more common by adolescence. It has been observed that beginning in adolescence there may be an elevated incidence of obesity. Microcephaly is reported in 10% (Digilio et al., 2001).

Table 3: Medical Problems with 22qDS

- Palatal anomalies (especially submucous cleft palate, velopharyngeal insufficiency)
- Hearing impairment
- Congenital heart defects
- Structural kidney anomalies
- Endocrine (especially hypoparathyroidism, hypothyroidism)
- Feeding/gastrointestinal problems
- Decreased platelet counts
- Immunological deficiencies and autoimmune disorders
- Neurological symptoms
- Scoliosis and other musculoskeletal problems

A thorough medical evaluation is essential once 22qDS has been diagnosed. See Table 3. A complete work-up for other associated medical features should be performed remembering that any organ system can be involved and that some features first present in adult years. See Table 4.

Table 4: Recommended Workup Once 22qDS Diagnosis Is Established

- Physical examination
- Developmental history
- Medical, surgical and psychiatric history
- Family history
- Genetic counselling for the patient and family
- FISH testing of parents for 22q11.2 deletion
- Blood work (recommended on an **annual** basis)

  Complete blood count including platelets

  Ionized calcium (note: different from serum calcium)

  Parathyroid hormone

Thyroid stimulating hormone

♦ Other investigations (if results not previously available)

Renal ultrasound

Echocardiogram

Specialist referrals as needed

Developmental/Cognitive Features

We are beginning to understand cognitive functioning in children with 22qDS but there are as yet few studies of adults. The work is ongoing. Some of the findings to date will be summarized.

Children with 22qDS are frequently described to have delayed motor and speech development and minor fine motor or coordination problems. A sample of 112 pre-school children (4 months to 6 years) was studied by a team at C.H.O.P. using standardized tests of language skills and general development (Gerdes et al., 2001). Of this group, 22% tested in an average range for cognitive development, but most showed developmental delay (24% mild delay, 54% significantly delayed in all areas of learning, i.e. cognition, motor, self help, languages). Severe and profound retardation were not seen in this sample. 80% were below average in language development. There were almost always delays in expressive speech. The majority had no speech at 2 years of age. There was no correlation between severity of developmental and intellectual delays and specific physical abnormalities such as cogenital heart defects. Voice quality disturbances, articulation errors, dysarthria and hypotonia were frequently observed. The authors suggested that attention should be given to early intervention tailored to the needs of each preschooler. This could include physical therapy for hypotonia, speech therapy, special instruction or occupational therapy (Gerdes et al., 2001).

Full scale I.Q. scores in 22qDS generally range from average to moderate mental retardation with average intellectual level usually reported in the low borderline range (Swillen et al., 2000). The prevalence of mental retardation is around 40% (Bassett et al., 1998; Goldberg et al., 1993). A recent study reported results of neuropsychological testing from 80 children, 50 of whom were school age (6 - 17 years) (Woodin et al., 2001). Two thirds had special educational support at school. However, replicating other studies (Swillen et al., 1997), verbal I.Q. exceeded performance or non-verbal I.Q. in a subset of children. The discrepancy between verbal and non-verbal reasoning abilities may be sufficiently severe to consider a diagnosis of non-verbal learning disability (NVLD) in a subset of children with 22qDS. It is important to note that those with 22qDS can have both receptive or expressive language difficulties as well as difficulties with non-verbal communication (Swillen et al., 2000).

Relative cognitive strengths in 22qDS include verbal skills, rote verbal learning and memory, reading and spelling. Weaknesses are often displayed in non-verbal processing or reasoning, visual-spatial skills and memory, complex verbal memory, mathematics, working memory, and attention (Swillen et al., 2000). As with all other features of 22qDS there is individual variability in cognitive test results. In general, educational planning should be aimed at developing the child's strengths and remediation for areas of weakness, based on a comprehensive assessment of each child's individual needs. Interactive computer-based learning programs have been useful children with 22qDS and effective in special education classroom settings (Kok & Solman, 1995).

Similar to findings in children, mean IQ in adults with 22qDS is in the low borderline range (Bassett et al., 1998; Chow, Watson, Young, Weksberg, & Bassett, 2002) varying from normal IQ with learning disabilities to, in rarer instances, severe mental retardation. The cognitive profile is also variable in adults and, overall, includes similar strengths and weaknesses to those found in children. The profile appears to differ in individuals who have schizophrenia (Chow et al., 2002). As with other forms of schizophrenia, those with 22qDS-schizophrenia have more severe weaknesses in verbal learning and recall (memory) (Chow et al., 2002).

Psychiatric Disorders Associated with 22qDS

Symptoms of emotional and/or behavioural disorder appear to be common in children with 22qDS and present a major source of concern for families. Specific psychiatric problems that have been identified include anxiety, emotional instability and disruptive behavioral disorders such as attention deficit / hyperactivity disorder (Goldberg et al., 1993; Niklasson, Rasmussen, Óskarsdóttir, & Gillberg, 2001; Swillen et al., 2000). There is some evidence that autistic-like features may be seen with moderate and severe mental retardation (Niklasson et al., 2001). Childhood behavioural concerns consistently found in elevated levels in 22qDS include social and attentional problems (Golding-Kushner, Weller, & Shprintzen, 1985; Swillen et al., 2000). Children are often described as either socially withdrawn or socially disinhibited with impulsivity (Golding-Kushner et al., 1985). Temper or emotional outbursts are common (Bassett et al., 1998). There have been reports of more anxiety and depression in adolescence (Swillen et al., 1999) that may be related to hormonal changes, increased academic and social demands or a genetic predisposition. Caregivers need to be providing appropriate supports and be vigilant for persistent changes in mood, thought or behaviour warranting referral to professional services knowledgeable about the disorder.

A number of researchers have reported a high frequency of psychiatric disorders associated with adolescents and adults with 22qDS (Bassett et al., 1998; Gothelf et al., 1997; Papolos et al., 1996; Pulver et al., 1994; Shprintzen, Goldberg, Golding-Kushner, & Marion, 1992). In an extensive review, Cohen et al. (1999) reported that 36% of adults with 22qDS had a psychiatric history, with many involving a psychotic illness; 64% had a psychiatric diagnosis if those ascertained as parents transmitting the deletion were excluded. In another study of 48 adults with a 22q11.2 deletion, 27% of the individuals had schizophrenia or schizoaffective disorder (Murphy, Jones, & Owen, 1999). Two patients had other psychotic illnesses, thus the prevalence of a psychotic illness was 30% in this sample, similar to that found in a previous study (Pulver et al., 1994). The age at onset of psychosis in 22qDS ranges from childhood to mid-40's (Bassett et al., 1998; Murphy et al., 1999). The clinical, structural brain, and cognitive profile of a 22qDS subtype of schizophrenia appears similar to that found in other forms of schizophrenia (Bassett, Chow, O'Neill, & Brzustowicz, 2001; Bassett et al., 2003).

The rate of schizophrenia in adults with 22qDS is clearly higher than either the general population (about 1%) or the developmentally delayed population (about 3%) (Turner, 1989). There does not appear to be evidence for such elevated rates of psychotic disorders in other genetic syndromes for which behavioural phenotypes have been described (Turk & Hill, 1995). Other psychiatric diagnoses found in adults with 22qDS include anxiety disorders, major depression, and alcoholism (Bassett, Chow, AbdelMalik, Gheorghiu, & Weksberg, 2003; Bassett et al., 1998; Cohen et al., 1999; Murphy et al., 1999; Pulver et al., 1994), although anxiety disorders appear to be particularly prevalent.

It is important to note that although many with 22qDS do not suffer from major psychiatric complications, accurate information will help caregivers to be more alert to early signs of these conditions and better able to secure necessary psychiatric and behavioural supports. As with other well-described syndromes, this understanding provides benefits such as a measure of control rather than helplessness, frustration, and guilt, which are so often experienced by caregivers (Turk & Sales, 1996).

Case Study #2

Sandy was born in the 1970's. She was delivered by cesarean section with fetal distress at 42 weeks gestation. Shortly after birth she was noted to have inspiratory stridor (a high-pitched, harsh sound when she breathed in) and feeding difficulties (gagging, coughing during feeds). Her parents were concerned that something was wrong but were offered no explanation. She was treated with an antibiotic for the cough.

At age 2-1/2 she was assessed by a speech pathologist. Although she was speaking in sentences, she was barely intelligible because of "air escaping through her nose" or hypernasal speech. A submucous cleft palate was identified. She subsequently had surgery to repair her palate and pharyngeal flap to reduce nasal air flow during speech.

She was enrolled in a preschool, then entered the public school system. She disliked school and the teasing she received about her speech. There had been efforts to keep her in a regular classroom setting with a reduced workload but this still created increasing frustration and an awareness that she could not keep up with others. At age 10 the parents were made aware of significant academic difficulties and were themselves witnessing a change in Sandy's emotional state. Sandy had become highly anxious and her distress was associated with vomiting. This persisted over several years. Gastrointestinal work-ups could find no organic cause for vomiting.

Sandy's parents recall that the start of high school was "too much for her." Over several years they noted an increase in bizarre and aggressive behavior to the point where Sandy became unmanageable at home. She became distressed and consumed by fears that strangers were staring at her and "doing things" to her. She complained of hearing voices telling her what to do. She had difficulties elaborating on these experiences or expressing her story in words to the numerous outpatient or inpatient psychiatrists, but would more often explode into outbursts of yelling or bouts of vomiting.

While she was on the psychiatric ward of a university hospital, she received a CT scan of the brain and EEG, which were unremarkable. She was treated with traditional antipsychotic medication, a behavior program and family interventions. A genetics consult was obtained and it was concluded that there was no obvious genetic basis to explain Sandy's problems. She was discharged from the psychiatric ward to an adolescent unit affiliated with the hospital and eventually to a series of group homes.

Ten years later Sandy was referred to an interdisciplinary team for the dually diagnosed because of ongoing problems with unshakable belief that strangers were watching/influencing her, episodes of uncontrollable agitation and poor response to caregiver's support measures. The team re-referred the family to genetics. There was no family history of developmental disability or major medical or psychiatric problems. On examination, her height was "on par" with family members. Apart from hypernasal speech, most striking physically were almond shaped eyes, flat cheekbones, a prominent nasal tip and slender, tapered fingers. A F.I.S.H. test was positive for 22q deletion syndrome. Her parents were negative for the deletion.

Once a genetic diagnosis was made and the syndrome explained by a genetic counsellor, the family expressed an enormous sense of relief at "finally having an answer." They had felt helpless and blamed, but now "we have it on paper...it's not our fault." They were further reassured through medical/neurological evaluations.

Care was informed by the literature on 22qDS. In particular, despite Sandy's difficulties describing to the psychiatrist details of her delusional and hallucinatory experiences, careful attention was paid to the observations of others across settings and psychosis was clearly evident. A treatment trial of a newer, atypical antipsychotic medication was initiated with marked improvement in thought processes and preoccupation with paranoid thoughts over a period of 1 year. Serotonin reuptake inhibitor treatment for persistent anxiety was also associated with a reduction in vomiting.

The family and group home worked with the teams' psychologist, speech pathologist and behavior therapist to identify areas of strength and weakness. Neuropsychological assessment placed her in the mild range of mental retardation. Her verbal I.Q. exceeded her non-verbal I.Q. and adaptive skills. Areas of strength included simple focused attention, rote verbal memory and word reading/decoding. Clear deficits were noted in language processing, working memory, complex verbal memory, executive functioning and emotional functioning. The team and caregivers were able to formulate suitable approaches for day to day interactions (e.g., slow rate of speech, short, simple phrases - much the way Sandy spoke), enhancing adaptive skills (e.g., step by step diagrams, supportive coaching/cueing, modeling and repetition), learning style in special educational classroom (e.g., computer used with good effect and enthusiasm) and ways to avoid or deal with stressful situations (e.g., outings with a suitable "coach", a quiet place to retreat if necessary). She also became an eager participant in social skills and anger management groups.

With multi-modal intervention and an integrated care approach Sandy's parents stress that they are now able to see their daughter for who she is —"a unique person with a personality all her own who wants to know she is loved."

Identifying Individuals Who May Have 22qDS

Screening criteria have been proposed to identify who should be tested for a 22q11.2. deletion (Bassett & Chow, 1999). Using these clinical criteria significantly enhanced the likelihood that an individual would be found to have 22qDS. Therefore, a thorough developmental, medical and psychiatric history, along with an awareness of dysmorphic features, is crucial to be able to decide whether consultation with a clinical genetics specialist should be sought and testing for a 22q11.2 deletion is warranted (Hodgkinson et al., 2001). See Table 5.

Table 5: Screening Criteria to Identify Adults at Increased Risk for 22q Deletion Syndrome[1]

Two or more of the following features[2]:

♦ Mental retardation (borderline to severe), learning difficulties

♦ Facial features: small ears, narrow palpebral fissures, prominent nose, retruded chin

♦ Hypernasal speech, velopharyngeal insufficiency, cleft palate (usually submucosal)

♦ Congenital heart defect: e.g., ventricular septal defect, tetralogy of Fallot

♦ Psychotic illness, schizophrenia, schizoaffective disorder

♦ History of hypocalcemia and/or hypoparathyroidism

♦ History of hypothymia (underdeveloped or absent thymus gland) or severe immune deficiency in infancy (rare)

Additional possible features:

♦ Other anomalies: e.g., asymmetric face (drooping of one side), talipes (club foot), polydactyly (extra finger or toe), kyphosis/ scoliosis, renal anomaly, hypospadias, patellar dislocations, hearing deficits

♦ Low platelet count (usually $<200 \times 10^9/l$)

♦ Any autoimmune disorder (e.g., hypothyroidism)

♦ Other psychiatric disorders (especially anxiety disorders) or behavioural features (e.g., emotional/temper outbursts)

♦ Family history of miscarriages, stillbirths, early infant deaths (rarely)

[1]*Adapted from Bassett & Chow, 1999 (Bassett & Chow, 1999).*

[2]*Clinical features in 22qDS are highly variable. Examples are provided of features reported in adults with schizophrenia (Bassett et al., 1998; Lazier et al., 2001). No single feature is found in all patients. Individual features are non-specific and may be found in many other conditions.*

Conclusion

22qDS is a common genetic syndrome that is present in the dually diagnosed patient population, particularly in individuals with psychotic illnesses and mild developmental delays. Clinical testing for the associated microdeletion on chromosome 22 has only been available since 1995. There is variable expression of congenital features, which may be subtle or corrected early in life, and these factors contribute to under-recognition of the syndrome, particularly in adults. Diagnosis of 22qDS has important genetic counselling implications for the patient and the family, and may significantly alter medical management. Treatable conditions that may appear later on in life include hypocalcemia which can predispose to seizures, and a variety of psychiatric illnesses. Developmental delays require educational and social supports based on a comprehensive assessment. 22qDS is the epitomy of a multisystem condition that requires a multidisciplinary team approach across all developmental stages.

Acknowledgments

Sincere thanks goes out to the individuals and families who have allowed us to tell their stories and use photographs. We are grateful to Drs. Jane Summers and Anthony Levinson for reviewing this project. Mention must be made of the work and time invested in the manuscript by Julia Ollinger and Mirona Gheorghiu.

Resources

Faces of Sunshine: The 22q11.2 Deletion A handbook for Parents and Professionals. Edited by Donna M. McDonald-McGinn, Brenda Finucane, Elaine Zackai.

Genetics and Mental Retardation Syndromes: A New Look at Behaviour and Interventions. Dykens, Hodapp, Finucane.

Genetics in Medicine: January/February 2001, Vol.3/Number 1 (Issue devoted to 22q11.2 Deletion Syndrome)

22q and You Centre (and newsletter)
The Clinical Genetics Centre
The Children's Hospital of Philadelphia
34th Street and Civic Center Boulevard
Philadelphia, PA 19104
E-mail:lunny@email.chop.edu

Dr. Anne Bassett & the Clinical Genetics Research Program
E-mail:cgrp@camh.net
Web site: www.cgrp.ca

Velo-Cardio-Facial Syndrome Education Foundation
Jacobson Hall, Room 707, University Hospital
750 East Adams Street
Syracuse, NY 13210
E-mail:vcfsef@hscsyr.edu
Web site: www.vcfsef.org

The 22q11.2 Group
P.O.Box 1302
MK13 OLZ, United Kingdom
E-mail:22q11.2@melcom.cix.co.uk
Web site: www.vcfs.net

OMIM – On-Line Mendelian Inheritance of Man
Web site: http://www.ncbi.nlm.nih.gov/omim/

NCBI Genes and Disease
Web site:www.ncbi.nlm.nih.gov/disease/DGS.html

GeneReviews
Web site: www.geneclinics.org

Linda Walters (Parental Support Group in Ontario)
27 Pinewood Avenue
Toronto, ON M6C 2V2 Canada
E-mail:eaflw@look.ca

References

Bassett, A. S., & Chow, E. W. C. (1999). 22q11 Deletion Syndrome: A genetic subtype of schizophrenia. *Biological Psychiatry, 46,* 882-891.

Bassett, A. S., Chow, E.W.C., AbdelMalik, P., Gheorghiu, M., Husted J., & Weksberg, R. (2003). The schizophrenia phenotype in 22q11 deletion syndrome. *American Journal of Psychiatry, 160*(9), 1580-1586.

Bassett, A. S., Chow, E. W. C., O'Neill, S., & Brzustowicz, L. (2001). Genetic insights into the neurodevelopmental hypothesis of schizophrenia. *Schizophrenia Bulletin, 27*(3), 417-430.

Bassett, A. S., Chow, E. W. C., & Weksberg, R. (2000). Chromosomal abnormalities and schizophrenia. *American Journal of Medical Genetics (Seminars in Medical Genetics), 97,* 45-51.

Bassett, A. S., Hodgkinson, K., Chow, E. W. C., Correia, S., Scutt, L. E., & Weksberg, R. (1998). 22q11 deletion syndrome in adults with schizophrenia. *American Journal of Medical Genetics (Neuropsychiatric Genetics), 81,* 328-337.

Boudjemline, Y., Fermont, L., Le Bidois, J., Lyonnet, S., Side, D., & Bonnet, D. (2001). Prevalence of 22q11 deletions in fetuses with conotruncal cardiac defects: a 6 year prospective study. *Journal of Pediatrics, 138*, 520-524.

Chow, E. W. C., Mikulis, D. J., Zipursky, R. B., Scutt, L. E., Weksberg, R., & Bassett, A. S. (1999). Qualitative MRI findings in adults with 22q11 Deletion Syndrome and schizophrenia. *Biological Psychiatry, 46*, 1436-1442.

Chow, E., Watson, M., Young, D., Weksberg, R., & Bassett, A. S. (2002). Neurocognitive profile of adults with 22q11.2 deletion Syndrome. *American Journal of Human Genetics. 71*, 265.

Chow, E. W. C., Zipursky, R. B., Mikulis, D. J., & Bassett, A. S. (2002). Structural brain abnormalities in patients with schizophrenia and 22q11 Deletion Syndrome. *Biological Psychiatry, 51*(3), 208-215.

Cohen, E., Chow, E. W. C., Weksberg, R., & Bassett, A. S. (1999). Phenotype of adults with the 22q11 Deletion Syndrome: A review. *American Journal of Medical Genetics, 86*, 359-365.

Demczuk, S., & Aurias, A. (1995). DiGeorge syndrome and related syndromes associated with 22q11.2 deletions: A review. *Annales de Genetique, 38*(2), 59-76.

Digilio, M. C., Marino, B., Cappa, M., Cambiaso, P., Giannotti, A., & Dallapiccola, B. (2001). Auxological evaluation in patients with DiGeorge/velocardiofacial syndrome (deletion 22q11.2 syndrome). *Genetics in Medicine, 3*(1), 30-33.

Driscoll, D. A., Salvin, J., Sellinger, B., Budarf, M. L., McDonald-McGinn, D. M., Zackai, E., et al. (1993). Prevalence of 22q11 microdeletions in DiGeorge and velocardiofacial syndromes: implications for genetic counselling and prenatal diagnosis. *Journal of Medical Genetics, 30*, 813-817.

Edelmann, L., Pandita, R. K., Spiteri, E., Funke, B., Goldberg, R., Palanisamy, N., et al. (1999). A common molecular basis for rearrangement disorders on chromosome 22q11. *Human Molecular Genetics, 8*(7), 1157-1167.

Eicher, P., McDonald-McGinn, D. M., Fox, C. A., Driscoll, D. A., Emanuel, B. S., & Zackai, E. H. (2000). Dysphagia in children with a 22q11.2 deletion: Unusual pattern found on modified barium swallow. *The Journal of Pediatrics, 137*(2), 158-164.

Eliez, S., Blasey, C. M., Schmitt, E. J., White, C. D., Hu, D., & Reiss, A. L. (2001). Velocardiofacial syndrome: Are structural changes in the temporal and mesial temporal regions related to schizophrenia? *American Journal of Psychiatry, 158*, 447-453.

Gerdes, M., Solot, C., Wang, P. P., McDonald-McGinn, D. M., & Zackai, E. H. (2001). Taking advantage of early diagnosis: Preschool children with the 22q11.2 deletion. *Genetics in Medicine, 3*(1), 40-44.

Goldberg, R., Motzkin, B., Marion, R., Scambler, P. J., & Shprintzen, R. J. (1993). Velo-cardio-facial syndrome: A review of 120 patients. *American Journal of Medical Genetics, 45,* 313-319.

Golding-Kushner, K. J., Weller, G., & Shprintzen, R. J. (1985). Velo-cardio-facial syndrome: Language and psychological profiles. *Journal of Craniofacial Genetics and Developmental Biology, 5,* 259-266.

Goldmuntz, E., Clark, B. J., Mitchell, L. E., Jawad, A. F., Cuneo, B. F., Reed, L., et al. (1998). Frequency of 22q11 deletions in patients with conotruncal defects. *Journal of the American College of Cardiology, 32*(2), 492-498.

Goodship, J., Cross, I., LiLing, J., & Wren, C. (1998). A population study of chromosome 22q11 deletions in infancy (original articles). *Archives of Disease in Childhood, 79*(4), 348-351.

Gothelf, D., Frisch, A., Munitz, H., Rockah, R., Aviram, A., Mozes, T., et al. (1997). Velocardiofacial manifestations and microdeletions in schizophrenic inpatients. *American Journal of Medical Genetics, 72,* 455-461.

Hall, J. G. (1993). CATCH 22. *Journal of Medical Genetics, 30,* 801-802.

Hodgkinson, K., Murphy, J., O'Neill, S., Brzustowicz, L., & Bassett, A. S. (2001). Genetic counselling for schizophrenia in the era of molecular genetics. *Canadian Journal of Psychiatry, 46,* 123-130.

Karayiorgou, M., Morris, M. A., Morrow, B., Shprintzen, R. J., Goldberg, R., Borrow, J., et al. (1995). Schizophrenia susceptibility associated with interstitial deletions of chromosome 22q11. *Proceedings of the National Academy of Sciences of the United States of America, 92,* 7612-7616.

Kelly, D., Goldberg, R., Wilson, D., Lindsay, E., Carey, A., Goodship, J., et al. (1993). Confirmation that the velo-cardio-facial syndrome is associated with haplo-insufficiency of genes at chromosome 22q11. *American Journal of Medical Genetics, 45,* 308-312.

Kok, L. L., & Solman, R. T. (1995). Velocardiofacial syndrome: Learning difficulties and intervention. *Journal of Medical Genetics, 32,* 612-618.

Lazier, K., Chow, E. W. C., AbdelMalik, P., Scutt, L., Weksberg, R., & Bassett, A. S. (2001). Low platelet count in 22q11 Deletion Syndrome and schizophrenia. *Schizophrenia Research, 50,* 177-180.

Lindsay, E. A. (2001). Chromosomal microdeletions: dissecting del22q11 syndrome. *Nature Reviews Genetics, 2,* 858-868.

Lindsay, E. A., Goldberg, R., Jurecic, V., Morrow, B., Carlson, C., Kucherlapati, R. S., et al. (1995). Velo-cardio-facial syndrome: Frequency and extent of 22q11 deletions. *American Journal of Medical Genetics, 57,* 514-522.

Lipson, A. H., Yuille, D., Angel, M., Thompson, P. G., Vandervoord, J. G., & Beckenham, E. J. (1991). Velocardiofacial (Shprintzen) syndrome: an important syndrome for the dysmorphologist to recognise. *Journal of Medical Genetics, 28,* 596-604.

McDonald-McGinn, D. M., Tonnesen, M. K., Laufer-Cahana, A., Finucane, B., Driscoll, D. A., Emanuel, B. S., et al. (2001). Phenotype of the 22q11.2 deletion in individuals identified through an affected relative: Cast a wide *FISH*ing net! *Genetics in Medicine, 3*(1), 23-29.

Mitnick, R. J., Bello, J. A., & Shprintzen, R. J. (1994). Brain anomalies in velo-cardio-facial syndrome. *American Journal of Medical Genetics (Neuropsychiatric Genetics), 54,* 100-106.

Murphy, K. C., Jones, L. A., & Owen, M. J. (1999). High rates of schizophrenia in adults with velo-cardio-facial syndrome. *Archives of General Psychiatry, 56,* 940-945.

Niklasson, L., Rasmussen, P., Óskarsdóttir, S., & Gillberg, C. (2001). Neuropsychiatric disorders in the 22q11 deletion syndrome. *Genetics in Medicine, 3*(1), 79-84.

Papolos, D. F., Faedda, G. L., Veit, S., Goldberg, R., Morrow, B., Kucherlapati, R., et al. (1996). Bipolar spectrum disorders in patients diagnosed with velo-cardio-facial syndrome: Does a hemizygous deletion of chromosome 22q11 result in bipolar affective disorder? *American Journal of Psychiatry, 153,* 1541-1547.

Pulver, A. E., Nestadt, G., Goldberg, R., Shprintzen, R. J., Morrow, B., Karayiorgou, M., et al. (1994). Psychotic illness in patients diagnosed with velo-cardio-facial syndrome and their relatives. *Journal of Nervous and Mental Disease, 182,* 476-478.

Ravnan, J. B., Chen, E., Golabi, M., & Lebo, R. V. (1996). Chromosome 22q11.2 microdeletions in velocardiofacial syndrome patients with widely variable manifestations. *American Journal of Medical Genetics, 66,* 250-256.

Ryan, A. K., Goodship, J. A., Wilson, D. I., Philip, N., Levy, A., Siedel, H., et al. (1998). Spectrum of clinical features associated with interstitial chromosome 22q11 deletions: A European collaborative study. *Journal of Medical Genetics, 34,* 798-804.

Scambler, P. J., Kelly, D., Lindsay, E., Williamson, R., Goldberg, R., Shprintzen, R., et al. (1992). Velo-cardio-facial syndrome associated with chromosome 22 deletions encompassing the DiGeorge locus. *Lancet, 339,* 1138-1139.

Scutt, L., Chow, E. W. C., Weksberg, R., Honer, W. G., & Bassett, A. S. (2001). Patterns of dysmorphic features in schizophrenia. *American Journal of Medical Genetics (Neuropsychiatric Genetics), 105,* 713-723.

Shprintzen, R. J., Goldberg, R., Golding-Kushner, K. J., & Marion, R. W. (1992). Late-onset psychosis in the velo-cardio-facial syndrome (letter). *American Journal of Medical Genetics, 42,* 141-142.

Shprintzen, R. J., Goldberg, R. B., Young, D., & Wolford, L. (1981). The velo-cardio-facial syndrome: a clinical and genetic analysis. *Pediatrics, 67*(2), 167-172.

Sullivan, K. E. (2001). DiGeorge syndrome/chromosome 22q11.2 deletion syndrome. *Current Allergy & Asthma Reports. 1,* 438-444.

Swillen, A., Devriendt, K., Legius, E., Eyskens, B., Dumoulin, M., Gewillig, M., et al. (1997). Intelligence and psychosocial adjustment in velocardiofacial syndrome: a study of 37 children and adolescents with VCFS. *Journal of Medical Genetics, 34,* 453-458.

Swillen, A., Devriendt, K., Legius, E., Prinzie, P., Vogels, A., Ghesquiere, P., et al. (1999). The behavioral phenotype in velo-cardio-facial syndrome (VCFS): from infancy to adolescence. *Genetic Counseling, 10,* 79-88.

Swillen, A., Vogels, A., Devriendt, K., & Fryns, J. P. (2000). Chromosome 22q11 deletion syndrome: Update and review of the clinical features, cognitive-behavioral spectrum, and psychiatric complications. *American Journal of Medical Genetics (Semin. Med. Genet.), 97,* 128-135.

Turk, J., & Hill, P. (1995). Behavioural phenotypes in dysmorphic syndromes. *Clinical Dysmorphology, 4,* 105-115.

Turk, J., & Sales, J. (1996). Behavioural phenotypes and their relevance to child mental health professionals. *Child Psychology and Psychiatry Review, 1,* 4-11.

Turner, T.H. (1989). Schizophrenia and mental handicap: A historical review, with implications for further research. *Psychological Medicine, 19,* 301-304.

Weinzimer, S. A. (2001). Endocrine aspects of the 22q11.2 deletion syndrome. *Genetics in Medicine, 3*(1), 19-22.

Wilson, D. I., Burn, J., Scambler, P., & Goodship, J. (1993). DiGeorge syndrome: part of CATCH 22. *Journal of Medical Genetics, 30,* 852-856.

Woodin, M., Wang, P. P., Aleman, D., McDonald-McGinn, D. M., Zackai, E. H., & Moss, E. (2001). Neuropsychological profile of children and adolescents with the 22q11.2 microdeletion. *Genetics in Medicine, 3*(1), 34-39.

CHAPTER 8

Angelman Syndrome

Jane Summers and Dianne Pittman

Introduction

In a 1965 paper, an English physician named Dr. Harry Angelman presented the details of three unrelated children who displayed a striking similarity to each other. All three children had abnormalities in the size and shape of their skull, severe seizure disorder, ataxic or jerky movements, severe developmental disability, lack of speech development, and frequent bouts of laughter. While the exact cause of their condition was unknown, Angelman asserted that it was the result of faulty embryological development.

In the years following the publication of Angelman's paper, several more accounts appeared describing children with similar clinical characteristics. The etiology of the syndrome (which eventually came to be known as Angelman syndrome or AS) remained unknown until 1987, when a microdeletion was discovered on the long arm of chromosome 15 (bands q11-q13) in several individuals with the characteristic clinical features (Kaplan, Wharton, Elias, Mandell, Donlon, & Latt, 1987; Magenis, Brown, Lacy, Budden, & LaFranchi, 1987). A deletion in a similar region of chromosome 15 had already been detected among individuals with Prader Willi syndrome (PWS). Thus, it was of great interest to scientists to find that two clinically distinct syndromes that were associated with developmental disability originated from a similar locus on chromosome 15. Soon after, a maternal origin for the AS deletion was discovered (Knoll, Nicholls, Magenis, Graham, Lalande, & Latt, 1989; Williams, Zori, Stone, Gray, Cantu, & Ostrer, 1990), in contrast to the finding that PWS is associated with a deletion on the paternal chromosome 15 (Butler & Palmer, 1983). This observation indicated that the parental origin of the deletion was a crucial factor. Thus, AS and PWS are reflective of the phenomenon known as genomic imprinting, in which certain genes may behave differently according to whether they are inherited from the mother or the father (Driscoll, 1994).

This chapter will begin by providing an overview of the genetic aspects of AS. This will be followed by an outline of the clinical features that are characteristic of the syndrome. Afterward, information regarding the cognitive, communication and behavioral profiles of individuals with AS will be shared. Case examples will be provided to illustrate clinical issues and outcomes. We will end by providing suggestions about future directions for intervention research.

Genetic Aspects of AS

Cause

While several genetic alterations or mechanisms are known to give rise to Angelman syndrome, they all basically result in the absence or inactivation of the maternally imprinted copy of what is believed to be the causative gene, the UBE-3A gene that is located on 15q11-q13. This gene encodes for the E6-AP protein, which is involved in a biochemical pathway that results in the breakdown of proteins that accumulate in the cytoplasm of cells in the body (Lombroso, 2000). Normally, the maternal copy of this gene is primarily active in the brain, while the paternal copy is almost completely inactive or "switched off" (this phenomenon is known as tissue specific imprinting). By contrast, both copies of the gene are switched on in the other organs and tissues in the body. Thus, the neurological features of AS are thought to be related in some way to the significant reduction in UBE-3A expression in the brain, since the maternal gene is not active or present in individuals with the syndrome and the paternal gene is naturally almost completely switched off (Rougeulle, Glatt, & Lalande, 1997). While the relative effects of reduced levels of UBE-3A gene expression on brain development and functioning are not clear (Jiang, Lev-Lehman, Bressler, Tsai, & Beaudet, 1999), cellular functions within the neurons are presumably disrupted (Lombroso, 2000). Apart from their severe neurological problems, individuals with AS are otherwise generally healthy since both paternal and maternal UBE-3A genes are expressed in other parts of the body.

Mechanisms

There are several ways in which the maternally imprinted copy of the UBE-3A gene can be disrupted. The most common reason is due to a large random or spontaneous interstitial deletion of maternal origin in the AS/PWS region of chromosome 15 (q11-q13). This deletion is very large when viewed at a molecular level (consisting of about 4 million base pairs) and results in the loss of several genes, including the critical UBE-3A gene as well as a pigment gene and a cluster of genes that are implicated in seizure disorders (Jiang, Lev-Lehman, Bressler, Tsai, & Beaudet, 1999). Deletion cases account for approximately 70% of all individuals with AS (Chan et al., 1993). (It should be noted that the percentages of individuals who fall into the different molecular categories may vary slightly from study to study). AS can also be caused by paternal uniparental disomy (UPD), in which both copies of chromosome 15 are inherited from the father (Malcolm et al., 1991). UPD cases are more rare, accounting for only about 3-4% of cases. In a third group of individuals, there is no maternal deletion of 15q11-q13 and copies of chromosome 15 are inherited from both parents. The maternal chromosome 15, however, carries a paternal imprint due to a defect in an imprinting control center. Consequently, the maternal copy of the UBE-3A gene functions like the paternal copy and is virtually silenced in the brain. Imprinting defects occur in about 6-10% of individuals with AS (Jiang et al., 1999). A small mutation has been detected in the maternally imprinted UBE-3A gene itself in a fourth group of individuals with AS, comprising about 4-6% of cases (Kishino, Lalande & Wagstaff, 1997). In the remaining group of individuals (about 10-14%), it is not possible to detect any molecular abnormalities of 15q11-q13. For them, a tentative diagnosis of AS is made on the basis of clinical history and features. There is the possibility that some as yet undiscovered mechanism is responsible for their AS, as well as the chance that they have been diagnosed incorrectly because another condition has given rise to clinical features that resemble the AS phenotype ("mimicking conditions"), such as a terminal deletion of 22q11.3 or duplication of 15q11-13 (Williams, Lossie, & Driscoll, 2001).

Prevalence

The prevalence of AS is estimated to be between approximately 1/12,000 to 1/20,000 births (Clayton-Smith & Pembrey, 1992; Steffenburg, Gillberg, Steffenburg, & Kyllerman, 1996). Among individuals with developmental disability and seizure disorder, however, the prevalence may be higher (Clayton-Smith, 1995), including adults with severe disability who live in long-term care facilities and who may have been overlooked (Buckley, Dinno, & Weber, 1998; Jacobsen, King, Leventhal, Christian, Ledbetter, & Cook, 1998). Depending upon the mechanism that causes the syndrome, the risk of recurrence is very small (less than 1%) or quite substantial (up to 50%). There are accounts of siblings having AS (Fisher, Burn, Alexander, & Gardner-Medwin, 1987; Willems, Dijkstra, Brouwer, & Smit, 1987). AS has been reported among different racial groups and in various countries around the world (Williams et al., 1995).

Testing

If an individual is suspected of having AS, guidelines that were established for diagnostic testing should be followed (American Society of Human Genetics, 1996). Genetic tests may be performed simultaneously or in a staged manner, depending upon the individual situation. Molecular testing using FISH (fluorescence in situ hybridization) can detect the presence of a deletion on 15q11-q13 and DNA methylation analysis can determine whether the deletion is of maternal origin. Methylation analysis can also detect whether the maternal chromosome 15 carries a paternal imprint (for cases involving imprinting defects) or whether the maternal chromosome 15 is missing (for UPD cases); additional testing is needed to confirm the underlying molecular mechanism in these two types of cases. Molecular tests for defects in the UBE-3A gene are now available but imprinting center molecular testing is not readily available. In some cases of proven AS, chromosome study using high resolution chromosome analysis may be necessary to identify translocation or other chromosomal rearrangements in the mother.

Why Is It Important To Know About the Genetic Mechanism?

There are at least two reasons why it is important to know about the underlying cause of AS in an individual. The first is that the risk of recurrence differs according to mode of inheritance. The lowest risk of recurrence (<1%) is found in deletion or UPD cases. A much higher risk of recurrence (up to 50%) can happen when mutations in the UBE-3A gene or imprinting center are inherited from the mother. An increased risk of recurrence is also present if AS is caused by an inherited chromosomal translocation. In cases where there are no molecular abnormalities, the recurrence risk is unknown but theoretically could be as high as 50%. Given this complex picture, it is easy to see why families need access to genetic counseling by professionals who are well acquainted with the rapidly evolving knowledge in regard to the genetics of AS.

The second reason why it is important to know about the underlying genetic mechanism is related to the finding of phenotypic differences among individuals with different etiologies for their AS. Individuals with AS that is caused by a deletion of 15q11-q13 have the most pronounced or classical physical and neurobehavioral abnormalities (Smith et al., 1996), while nondeletion cases that are caused by UPD or involve mutations in the UBE-3A gene or imprinting center typically have a somewhat less severe phenotype (Bottani et al., 1994; Moncla et al., 1999a; Moncla et al., 1999b). Moncla et al. (1999b) have proposed ordering the molecular classes on a gradient of clinical severity (from most severe to least severe), such that deletion cases > UBE-3A mutations > imprinting defects and/or UPD cases. Advances in knowledge have resulted in a growing recognition that the clinical features of AS may be more heterogeneous than once thought. Thus, identification of a broader spectrum of AS features has important implications for diagnosis, prognosis and treatment.

Physical and Neurodevelopmental Features of AS

The clinical characteristics of AS have been divided into three categories: those that are consistently present (100% of cases), frequent features (80%) and associated features (20-80%). The following information has been obtained from the diagnostic consensus criteria that were developed by Williams et al. (1995).

The universal features of AS are developmental disability (functionally severe range), ataxic or jerky motor movements, absent or minimal expressive speech and relatively better receptive language, happy demeanor with frequent bouts of laughter, hyperactivity and short attention span. Seizures (onset usually before age 3), abnormal EEG patterns, and delayed growth in head circumference are frequently present. Associated features may be more variable in their expression and frequency. These include a range of cranio-facial and oro-motor characteristics, including flat occiput (back of head), protruding tongue and tongue thrusting, wide mouth and widely spaced teeth, and prominent jaw. Arms may be uplifted and hands held in a flexed position while walking. Feeding problems during infancy may occur, and excessive drooling and mouthing or chewing objects has been noted. Sleep disturbance has been documented as well.

As mentioned previously, the frequency and severity of clinical characteristics varies among the different molecular classes of AS. A comparison of features in deletion and nondeletion cases is presented in Table 1.

Table 1. Phenotypic Differences Between Deletion and Nondeletion Cases[a]

Deletion Cases	Nondeletion Cases[b]
♦ microcephaly in 90%, present by age 2 ♦ seizure disorder present in almost 100%, usually developing before 3 years of age ♦ growth retardation in 50%, obesity in 15% of cases ♦ ~75-80% walk independently beginning ~ 5 years of age on average ♦ hypopigmentation in 75% of cases ♦ minimal expressive speech (about 2 words) ♦ poor at using non-verbal forms of communication ♦ require assistance with activities of daily living as adolescents and adults	♦ microcephaly in ~1/3 of cases ♦ seizure disorder in ~ 70%, usually developing around 5 years of age ♦ growth retardation in 10% and obesity in 50% of cases ♦ all learn to walk independently beginning ~2 ½ years of age on average ♦ no cases of hypopigmentation ♦ expressive speech somewhat better (4 to 20+ words) ♦ relatively better non-verbal communication skills ♦ more independent with activities of daily living as adolescents and adults

[a] *Derived from Moncla, Malzac, Voelckel et al. (1999b); Smith et al. (1996)*

[b] *Consists of UPD, imprinting defects, and UBE-3A gene mutations*

Natural History of AS

Birth and Infancy

Following what is usually an uncomplicated pregnancy and delivery, the earliest manifestations of AS are non-specific, including feeding problems (related to weak suck and swallow, tongue thrusting, regurgitation, reflux) and poor weight gain, hypotonia and jerky limb movements (Fryburg, Breg, & Lindren, 1991; Van Lierde, Atza, Giardino, & Viani, 1990; Yamada & Volpe, 1990). Reduced cooing and babbling may be noted, and seizures may develop before one year of age in a percentage of infants. Parents typically seek a medical evaluation in response to one or more of these concerns (Zori, Hendrickson, Woolven, Whidden, Gray, & Williams, 1992), and a diagnosis of failure-to-thrive, cerebral palsy or global developmental delay may be given (e.g., Wilcox, 1991). Prader-Willi may be mistakenly diagnosed on the basis of developmental delay, feeding problems and hypotonia, but the dissimilarity of the two syndromes becomes more obvious over time. Part of the difficulty in making the diagnosis of AS in infants and very young children is that the characteristic cranio-facial and behavioral features are not very pronounced. As time goes by, however, these features evolve more fully and become more distinctive. Key aspects of AS at different ages are noted in Table 2.

Childhood

Generally, the course of development in children with AS is typified by severely limited but forward progression in skills (information on children's cognitive, communication and behavioral profiles will be presented in subsequent sections). While most children with AS do eventually learn to walk, the timing of when this occurs is influenced by the extent of their gait and movement disorder. Children with more severe balance and coordination problems learn to walk later and display movement patterns that are characteristic of AS (e.g., wide-based stance, arms held up and hands pointing forward and down). Many but not all children have light-colored hair, skin and eyes.

Seizure disorder is usually evident by 5 years of age. For many children, seizures are difficult to control initially, and different medications may be tried until optimal control is achieved. During the early-to-mid school years, skill development and behavior management issues seem to take center stage. Problems with children's reduced levels of sleep, high levels of motor activity, and extremely short attention span may place inordinately high demands on caregivers to provide constant supervision and assistance with activities of daily living. While these factors may combine to make this a particularly challenging period of time, the situation may be offset by children's sociability and pleasant disposition.

Table 2. Natural History of AS[a]

Age	Characteristics
Infancy and early childhood	◆ feeding problems ◆ jerky movements, poor muscle tone ◆ abnormal EEG pattern; seizures may develop ◆ developmental delays ◆ absent or delayed babbling ◆ happy disposition ◆ physical growth parameters may start to slow down ◆ sleep problems may be present
Middle childhood	◆ seizures develop in most by age 5 but tend to become milder and easier to control over time ◆ microcephaly is present in many ◆ facial features evolve (prominent jaw, wide mouth and widely spaced teeth) ◆ most will be walking by age 5 ◆ hyperactivity and reduced attention span are very noticeable ◆ sleep disturbance may worsen ◆ severe expressive speech delays; somewhat better receptive language ◆ increased weight gain possible
Adolescence	◆ puberty is normal but onset may be delayed ◆ seizure picture may improve ◆ weight gain and obesity may occur ◆ mobility may decline in individuals with severe ataxia or those with weight gain ◆ scoliosis may develop during adolescent growth spurt or worsen ◆ sleep may improve
Adulthood	◆ generally healthy, normal life-span ◆ facial features are pronounced ◆ biggest issues are seizures and reductions in mobility with associated skeletal problems ◆ normal problems with aging ◆ happy disposition continues ◆ quieter and calmer, improved attention span, improvement in sleep ◆ variability in self-care skills but supervision still needed

[a]*Compiled from Buckley, Dinno & Weber (1998); Clayton-Smith (1993, 2001); Laan et al.(1996); Sandanam et al. (1997); Williams, Zori et al. (1995); Zori et al. (1992)*

Case Example 1: Christine

Christine is a 4 ½ -year-old girl with AS. She displays many of the features that are commonly reported among children and adults with AS – i.e., happy demeanor with frequent bouts of laughter, unsteady, broad-based gait with arms and hands flexed up, excessive physical contact (grabbing, pulling hair) and sleep disturbance. She was diagnosed at around 22 months of age by DNA methylation study and FISH analysis and was found to have a microdeletion of chromosome 15q11-q13. In regard to her early history, Christine was born following an uncomplicated pregnancy and delivery. During infancy, she was diagnosed with gastroesophageal reflux and failure-to-thrive. Although Christine's early milestones were delayed (she sat at 10 months and crawled at 15 months), her parents became very concerned by the fact that she was not walking or starting to speak by 18 months and sought specialized medical evaluation. She had jerking movements prior to 18 months but did not have clear seizures until age 4. Apart from a seizure disorder, Christine does not have any other medical problems.

Christine has undergone numerous developmental assessments. At the age of 21 months, she demonstrated skills at an age equivalent level of approximately 8-10 months. Her strengths were in the area of social responsiveness, exploration of the environment and gross motor skills, while expressive language was an obvious weakness. Further assessments were conducted when she was 26 months of age. At this time, her gross motor skills were determined to be at an age equivalent level of 10 months overall. A language assessment revealed that Christine demonstrated early intentional communication skills and an understanding of some single words within the context of daily routines. She learned to walk by 3 ½ years of age after intensive physiotherapy.

By 4 ½ years of age, Christine has made gains in all developmental realms. She is able to bring a spoon to her mouth but not scoop food. She can follow one-step directions in context and demonstrates understanding of some single signs. She can communicate her needs by leading people to what she wants. She has begun to point to desired objects and use pictures to communicate. She has started to vocalize more and may whine if her mother doesn't understand what she wants or if a desired object is not available or is taken away.

Christine's attention span is typically brief but she can sit for up to 30 minutes to watch a preferred television show. She is able to play with simple cause and effect toys but does not do so independently. Her seizure disorder is well-controlled and her sleep is greatly improved on melatonin. Her parents are concerned, however, about her tendency to grab and pull at other children who can become afraid of her. While her happy demeanor is protective in that people attribute her behavior to playfulness, her mother is concerned that as Christine gets older these behaviors will severely limit her social interactions and quality of life. The current approach to managing her excessive physical contact is to show her how to touch gently and to pair this with a verbal prompt to do so. Christine's family and staff are also working to improve her life skills in the areas of self-feeding and toileting.

Adolescence

Adolescence may bring some improvements but along with it new challenges. Seizures may become more infrequent in some adolescents with AS to the point where medication is no longer needed. Reductions in levels of motor activity and improvements in attention span have been noted (Clayton-Smith, 2001), along with increased sleep. Skills continue to develop and the process may be assisted by an improved ability to concentrate. Puberty often occurs at the typical time and females with AS are capable of reproduction (Lossie & Driscoll, 1999). Masturbation may become an issue but individuals can be directed to engage in this behavior in private. However, individuals with AS are very vulnerable to sexual exploitation due to their low level of intellectual functioning and sociable nature, and therefore require close supervision (Clayton-Smith, 2001).

Weight gain may become an issue during adolescence. Clayton-Smith (2001) reported that approximately one-third of adolescents and young adults with AS that were studied had become obese as teenagers, and that the majority of these individuals were females. Obesity in general was related to reductions in mobility and level of motor activity. Scoliosis may became evident during a period of rapid growth during the teenage years.

Adulthood

Most adults with AS are generally healthy and do not appear to have a reduced lifespan. Their happy disposition is still obvious, but they can and do show signs of sadness as well. Improvements in attention span and a reduction in hyperactivity have been noted in many individuals. There is no evidence of regression in skills and ongoing instruction in communication and self-care skills remains indicated. The major issues during this period continue to be related to seizures and problems with ambulation. Most adults with AS continue to experience seizures; however, the seizure type and frequency is variable. In one review, seizure control improved in about 40% of adults being studied and worsened in about 15-30% (Buckley, Dinno, & Weber, 1998; Clayton-Smith, 2001; Laan, Th. den Boer, Hennekam, Renier, & Brouwer, 1996; Sandanam, Beange, Robson, Woolnough, Buchholz, & Smith, 1997). In a proportion of the latter group, seizures recommenced after a relatively quiet period during adolescence and were difficult to bring under control. Mobility tends to deteriorate with age, in association with scoliosis and movement disorder. Some adults with AS require wheelchairs for safety reasons and to make it easier to care for their needs (Buckley et al., 1998).

A number of medical issues may arise which are not specifically associated with AS but are common to individuals with severe developmental disability and/or a result of the aging process (Buckley et al., 1998). These include cataracts, fractures due to falls, hypothyroidism, and diabetes. Clayton-Smith (2001) pointed out that esophageal reflux is common in adults with AS and can be severe in some cases.

Case Example 2: Ben

Ben is a 31-year-old male with AS. He was diagnosed by DNA test and FISH analysis (del 15q11q13) at the age of 26. In terms of his early history, he was very irritable and cried constantly. He had feeding problems (recurrent vomiting) as a young infant that eventually resolved. He developed seizures around one year of age. His parents became concerned about his development when he was 4 months of age. His developmental milestones were delayed – he crawled at 2 ½ years, stood alone at 4 years, and walked with an unsteady gait and arms and hands flexed up around 4 ½ years. He did not sleep more than a few hours a night and would often get up and destroy his mattress and furniture. As Ben became older, his parents had increasing difficulty managing his behavior and coping with the demands of their growing family. As a consequence, he was placed in a specialized behavior management unit at age 7. While at the unit, staff worked on skill development (toilet training and increasing his attention span) and decreasing inappropriate behaviors (aggression, tantrums and noncompliance). He was transferred into a long-term care facility where he remained until moving into a group home in the community near his parents at age 24.

Ben was referred to a specialized mental health service for adults with developmental disabilities at the age of 26. The presenting problems consisted of sleep disturbance, hyperactivity and excitability with excessive physical contact (hugs, grabs, pulling hair). He underwent an interdisciplinary assessment involving psychiatry, speech-language pathology and behavior therapy. The psychiatrist suspected he had AS and referred him to clinical genetics for a diagnostic assessment. Another aspect of the psychiatric consultation was to review the medications he had been taking for seizures, sleep disturbance and behavioral dyscontrol. The speech-language pathologist conducted a swallowing assessment because of an increase in Ben's coughing and choking at mealtimes. Recommendations were provided for modifications to his diet and for staff to monitor his portion size and rate of eating and drinking. Communication goals were established for Ben which consisted of helping him to make choices about activities, food items and articles of clothing to wear; to request help with toileting; and to increase his communication abilities in relation to routine events and activities. The behaviour therapist conducted an assessment to determine the function of Ben's inappropriate behaviour and worked with staff to develop a plan to increase the amount of structure and consistency in the home.

Over the next two years Ben's behavior worsened. He became overexcited by the presence of certain female staff and would lunge and grab at them constantly. At times he would cry when they left the area. There were days when he would stay on the couch for hours as well. Staff ratings on the Aberrant Behavior Checklist showed a major increase in scores on the scales that measured irritability, lethargy and social withdrawal, stereotypy and hyperactivity/noncompliance. Staffing and environmental issues were occurring around the same time that may have impacted Ben's behavior, as two new residents with challenging behavior moved into the home without an accompanying increase in staffing. Several measures were taken subsequently to deal with the situation. Staffing levels in the home were enhanced and new staff were hired who did not have a history with Ben and could get off to a fresh start with him. The new staff visited a group home that specialized in individuals with AS and obtained practical information as well as a more balanced perspective of their behavior. Staff provided more structured activities that were geared to Ben's interests and developmental level, including regular access to a stimulation room that contained gross motor and cause-and-effect items. They also permitted Ben to engage in limited physical contact, whereas they had previously discontinued all touching when he became aggressive. Efforts were made to address the needs of all the residents in the group home, which resulted in a quieter and more predictable environment. About a year later the discovery was made that Ben had major dental problems, which resulted in numerous cavities being filled and the removal of several teeth. It is likely that these dental problems had been undetected for some time. Unfortunately, the behavioral tracking was not done consistently throughout this period so it was not possible to determine the impact of different factors on Ben's behavior. A year later, Ben's behavior had settled remarkably and his ABC scores had dropped to within a more "typical range" for individuals with AS (Summers & Feldman, 1999). At present (3 years after the initial referral), Ben is able to sit and feed himself independently using a spoon. He can also sit for up to 10 minutes with staff and look through the pages of a photo album. He is going home for short visits and is not "mauling" people nearly as much as before. He is healthy although a bit thin. He has no problems with ambulation and is very active. His ABC scores remain within the a typical range for individuals with AS.

Treatment Issues

In general, the major health-related issues that are faced by individuals with AS are in relation to their seizure disorder and musculoskeletal problems. The medical management of seizures is an ongoing issue and the process is apt to be very active at times, particularly when seizures first emerge or become more difficult to manage. Orthopedic problems can also have a major impact on the quality of life of individuals with AS. Treatment options may consist of exercise, adaptive walking devices and bracing and/or surgery for scoliosis. Physiotherapy can be very important during various periods in time to assist the child with AS to learn to walk, encourage the adolescent with AS to remain active to prevent excessive weight gain and maintain a full range of motion, and to help the adult with AS to stay mobile as long as possible to guard against future joint and spine problems (Buckley et al., 1998; Clayton-Smith, 2001). Individuals with scoliosis may be at heightened risk for cardiorespiratory problems (Buntinx et al., 1995).

Other medical problems that have been reported among some individuals with AS include ocular/vision problems (particularly strabismus) and hearing difficulties caused by ear infections (Clayton-Smith, 1993; Zori et al., 1992). Reflux and gastrointestinal difficulties (Clayton-Smith, 1993) and obesity (Clayton-Smith, 2001) may also occur. Individuals with hypopigmentation are at risk of sunburn and protective measures such as sunscreen should be taken when going outside (Williams et al., 1995b).

Cognitive Development

As with many aspects of AS, there appears to be greater variability in cognitive abilities than was once thought. On a functional level, however, individuals with AS invariably have severe adaptive impairment. While the evidence for this statement is based on the results of developmental testing and clinical observation, it is important to recognize that findings can be affected by problems that are inherent in individuals with AS, such as lack of speech development, motor impairments, short attention span and hyperactivity.

Piaget's theory of intellectual development has been utilized by researchers to study the cognitive abilities of children and adults with AS. According to this theory, typically developing children between the ages of 0-24 months progress through a series of six stages within the "sensorimotor" period of cognitive development (this time period roughly corresponds with the cognitive level of individuals with AS). During the sensorimotor period, children's mental development is rooted in the organization and coordination of sensory and perceptual input with motor movements and actions (Yussen & Santrock, 1982). Over time, the infant's and toddler's behavior becomes progressively more systematic, goal-directed and, ultimately, inventive. By the end of the sensorimotor period (at approximately 2 years of age), the transition to symbolic thought is beginning to occur and language development proceeds (Ginsburg & Opper, 1979).

Penner, Johnston, Faircloth, Irish, and Williams (1993) used a Piagetian approach to assess different aspects of sensorimotor cognition in seven individuals with AS ranging in age from 12-40 years. All seven had previously been assessed to be functioning within the profound range of developmental disability on formalized measures and they all resided in an institution. Two notable findings emerged from this study. First, the level of cognitive abilities varied both within and among the participants, sometimes to a surprising degree. One participant in particular demonstrated some relatively advanced abilities within the sensorimotor period, corresponding to Stages 5-6 (12-24 months). Since there was no information regarding the molecular classification of the participants, it is not known whether this represented a non-deletion case. The second important finding was in regard to participants' consistently lowered levels of ability in the area of vocal and gestural imitation (with the exception of the same, less impaired participant who performed better in the area of gestural imitation than in the area of vocal imitation).

In a second study, Andersen, Rasmussen, and Stromme (2001) also used a Piagetian model to evaluate cognitive functioning in 20 children with AS, ranging in age from 2 to 14 years. In terms of underlying etiologies, 55% had a confirmed deletion of 15q11-q13, 10% had UPD, and 35% had received a diagnosis based on clinical features.

In general, children demonstrated highest levels of mastery on locomotor tasks (median level of performance corresponding to sensorimotor Stages 5-6) and lowest levels of mastery on tasks that required more complex and abstract thinking abilities (Stages 3-4). There was wide variation in individual performance, both within and across tasks, ranging from a low of 6 months to a high of 24 months. Six children, for instance, were observed to engage in constructive play with a ball or toy car; seven were able to imitate simple play; four were able to put together puzzles with shapes; and five looked at and turned the pages of a picture book It would be worthwhile to explore children's cognitive profiles in relation to their underlying molecular classification.

The results of these studies indicate that a number of children and adults with AS appear to have attained some of the cognitive prerequisites that underlie speech and language development. Thus, severe cognitive impairment alone is not accepted as the sole explanation for the striking deficits in communication that are a core feature of AS. These issues will be explored further in the section on communication development.

Adaptive Skills

Adaptive skills refer to activities that an individual performs in major life areas, including expressive and receptive communication, personal and domestic care, socialization, play and leisure, and motor tasks. Despite the availability of standardized assessment measures, it does not appear that adaptive functioning in individuals with AS has been studied in a formal manner. The little information that does exist is primarily descriptive in nature and is summarized in Table 3.

Table 3. Adaptive Functioning in Individuals With AS

Study and details	Findings
Smith et al. (1996) ♦ children to adults (3-34 years) ♦ all had deletions	♦ teenagers and adults were all dependent on assistance with feeding, toileting and dressing
Moncla, Malzac, Voelckel et al., (1999b) ♦ teenagers and adults (15-36 years) ♦ compared deletion to non-deletion cases	♦ vast majority of individuals with deletions were dependent on assistance for feeding, toileting and dressing ♦ majority of non-deletion cases did not need assistance for dressing and feeding
Clayton-Smith (2001) ♦ teenagers and adults (16-40 years) ♦ 68% had deletions	♦ all needed supervision ♦ 71% could self-feed ♦ 71% remained dry during the day and 89% needed diapers at night ♦ 61% could carry out basic household tasks ♦ 50% could dress/undress with simple fastenings on clothing
Laan et al. (1996) ♦ adults (20-53 years) ♦ 82% had deletions	♦ 85% could perform a simple task such as holding a utensil ♦ 50% helped to undress themselves ♦ 57% remained dry during the day (clock trained) and 11% overnight
Sandanam et al. (1997) ♦ adults (24-36 years) ♦ all had deletions	♦ all were dependent for activities of daily living

As with other aspects of AS, adaptive functioning may be somewhat higher among individuals who do not have a deletion. Standardized, quantifiable information is greatly needed in order to: (1) track the rate and quality of skill development over time; (2) assist in the selection of developmentally appropriate target skills and to evaluate the impact of intervention efforts; (3) permit a precise comparison of skills across different molecular categories within AS; and (4) compare skill levels in AS to different genetic syndromes.

Communication Development

Speech and Language

As mentioned in previous sections, one of the universal features of AS is absent or minimal speech and relatively better receptive language skills. While this observation appears in virtually all case reports of individuals with AS, only a handful of studies provide quantifiable information about their expressive and receptive language abilities (see Table 4) and seek to identify some of the factors that may limit their language development.

Expressive speech, when it does develop, consists of single word utterances. The maximum number of words that have been reported for any one individual is about 15-20 (Alvares & Downing, 1998; Moncla et al., 1999b). Words are often approximations and are difficult to understand. Despite varying degrees of success with speech and non-verbal forms of communication, expressive abilities are extremely delayed and fall well within the sensorimotor period of cognitive development, primarily at Stages 3-4 (up to 12 months) (Andersen, Rasmussen, & Stromme, 2001), when symbolic understanding and recognition of words are starting to emerge. Two separate studies (Jolleff & Ryan, 1993; Andersen et al., 2001) established an upper limit of 14 months when a parent report measure was used to evaluate expressive language abilities in children aged 2-15 years. There was, however, wide variability in individual children's scores, ranging from a low of 3 months to a high of 14 months.

Receptive language skills are relatively better developed in individuals with AS, although still very delayed. Returning to the previous studies, Andersen et al. (2001) reported a range of 5-24 months in age-equivalent scores among the children in their study when parental input was used to measure their receptive language functioning. Abilities at this upper limit of 24 months are sufficient for understanding simple instructions. The maximum gap between children's expressive and receptive functioning (in favor of the latter) was 10 months. Jolleff and Ryan (1993) assessed a comparable group of children and reported remarkably similar findings. Children's receptive language scores ranged from 9-22 months and their receptive language ability was always equal to or better than their expressive language ability (maximum difference of 11 months between the two). In both studies, children's mean receptive language scores were significantly better than their mean expressive language scores.

Table 4. Studies on Language Functioning in Children and Adults With AS

Author and year	Number of participants and age range	Study methods	Expressive language[a]	Receptive language
Jolleff & Ryan (1993)	11 children (range 2- 15 years)	parent interview	REEL[b] age equivalent scores -5/11 > 12 months (range 6-14 months)	REEL 7/11 > 12 months (range 9-22 months)
Summers et al. (1995)	108 cases (1 - 33 years)	meta analysis of published cases	of the 23 cases with sufficient detail: -words: 7/23 (range 1 - several words) -gestures: 3/23 -signs: 4/23	of the 9 cases with sufficient detail: -9/9 could understand simple commands or conversation
Summers et al. (1995)	11 children (1 - 12 years)	parent survey	.-babbles: 7/11 -words: 2/11 (range 1-3 words) -gestures: 9/11 -AAC: 4/11	-10/11 could follow simple instructions
Alvares & Downing (1998)	20 children (1 - 13 years)	parent survey	-vocalises: 20/20 -words: 11/20 (range 1-15 words) -signs: 10/20 (range 2 -200+ signs) -augmentative: 13/20 -pictures: 10/13 -voice output: 8/13	not studied
Anderson, Rasmussen & Stromme (2001)	20 children (2-14 years)	-standardised assessment -parent interview	REEL-2 age equivalent scores -6/20 > 12 months (median 8 months; range 3-14 months) direct assessment -words: 2/20 used 4-5 7/20 used 2-3 11/20 used 0-1 -signs or pictures: 6/20	REEL-2 -11/20 > 12 months (median 12 months; range 5-24 months)

[a] *Refers to emerging as well as developed skills*

[b] *Test of Receptive - Expressive Emergent Skills (REEL)*

Penner et al. (1993) assessed prelinguistic communication behavior in 7 children and adults with AS ranging in age from 12-40 years. None of them were able to produce speech or signs.The two most able individuals routinely used primitive (e.g., leading others to what s/he wanted) and conventional (e.g., pointing and gestures) intentional expressive communication behaviors. Four individuals were considered to be non-intentional communicators but could produce some primitive intentional behaviors when enticed to do so. The remaining individual could not be motivated to produce any intentional communication behaviors. Joint attention abilities were also studied among this group of individuals. Only one individual was able to use joint attention to sustain a social interaction; this individual also displayed the most advanced repertoire of conventional prelinguistic communication behaviors.

Augmentative and alternative communication (AAC)

Augmentative and alternative communication (AAC) approaches are proving to be a viable option for individuals with AS who are unable to acquire spoken language skills or as a means to enhance expressive abilities in those who have some minimal speech skills. Different examples of AAC approaches include manual signs, tangible symbols (real objects, miniature objects), representational symbols (photographs, picture communication symbols), and high and low technology devices (e.g., voice output systems, picture boards). Selection of appropriate AAC approaches should be guided by consideration of several factors, including the individual's current skills and communication needs, ability to use symbols, functional limitations (motor, visual or hearing impairments), and the preferences, skills and attitudes of their caregivers and other communication partners (Beukelman & Mirenda, 1992).

Only a few studies contain specific information about AAC usage by individuals with AS; these studies are summarized in Table 4. Several approaches have been used, including signs, picture systems, and voice output devices. Since these studies are primarily descriptive in nature, there is little or no information regarding how and when these approaches were introduced and how successful they are. Nonetheless, it is probably fair to say that AAC offers far greater promise as a means to enable individuals with AS to communicate in a functional manner than speech-based approaches alone.

Factors that limit language development

A developmental explanation alone is not considered to be sufficient to account for the disproportionately severe expressive language deficits that are characteristic of AS (Penner et al., 1993). Several factors may underlie individuals' low level of skill development (including language), while others may contribute more specifically to expressive language deficits. Examples of factors that impact on the learning performance and language development of individuals with AS include the following: presence of seizures and effects of anticonvulsant medication; vision (strabismus) and hearing (middle ear infections) problems; attentional difficulties and hypermotoric behavior; motor impairments; problems in initiating and maintaining joint attention; deficits in vocal and gestural imitation; abnormal or absent babbling or vocal play; and the presence of interfering behaviors (e.g., self-stimulatory behavior).

Some researchers have proposed a link between oral motor dysfunction and the severe expressive speech deficits that are characteristic of individuals with AS, citing the following factors:

♦ orofacial abnormalities that may affect oral function (prominent jaw, wide mouth and widely spaced teeth, protruding tongue)

♦ problems with planning and initiating motor acts (including speech), as evidenced by oro-motor and vocal imitation deficits; drinking, feeding and swallowing problems; problems with saliva control (drooling)

♦ lack of babbling and vocalizations

♦ nasal or guttural voice quality

♦ oral behaviors such as mouthing of objects

♦ movement disorders (e.g., ataxia, tremulousness) which may affect non-verbal modes of expressive communication, such as sign and gesture, as well as the ability to use AAC approaches that require a motor response

(Alvares, 2000; Alvares & Downing, 1998; Andersen et al., 2001; Jolleff & Ryan, 1993; Penner et al., 1993)

Behavioral Characteristics

One of the most striking and as a consequence frequently cited behavioral characteristics of individuals with AS is their "happy" demeanor. This apparent happiness is manifested by frequent laughter or smiling and a pleasant facial expression. Bouts of sadness and crying do occur as well (e.g., Laan et al., 1996) but may be overshadowed by the appearance of happiness. Displays of laughter and happiness have been referred to as inappropriate, excessive or unprovoked. A study by Oliver, Demetriades, and Hall (2002), however, illustrates that the occurrence of smiling and laughing is influenced by social-environmental events. Three children with AS (ranging in age from 7-17 years) participated in their study. Durations of children's smiling and laughing were highest when an adult provided continuous social praise; at intermediate levels when an adult sat nearby but did not interact or else engaged in instructional tasks with the child; and at lowest levels when the adult left the room. The findings indicate that even behaviors that may be related to an underlying genetic abnormality can be shaped and modified by environmental influences.

Other salient behavioral features consist of hyperactivity, attentional deficits and an excitable personality. This specific pattern of behavior is considered one of the key diagnostic criteria for AS, while an attraction to or fascination with water is listed as an associated diagnostic feature (Williams et al., 1995a). A more extensive list of behavioral correlates has been compiled by several researchers (e.g., Hersh et al.,

1981; Summers, Allison, Lynch, & Sandler, 1995; Zori et al., 1992). Summers et al. (1995) gathered systematic data on the nature and prevalence of behavior problems among individuals with AS. In the first part of the study, a meta analysis was conducted of 34 published case reports that involved 108 individuals. The behavioral concerns that were identified (in addition to speech deficits and laughter) in descending order of occurrence were: hyperactivity or restlessness; feeding problems as an infant; attention deficits; aggression; repetitive or stereotyped behavior; chewing or mouthing hands/objects; sleep problems; tantrums and noncompliance. In the second part of the study, the parents of eleven children with AS (ranging in age from 1-12 years) completed a standardized behavioral rating instrument. All eleven children were rated as being extremely restless and having problems maintaining their attention and concentration. "Aggressive" behavior was also reported among all eleven children; however, they were described as being more likely to grab at people and things than to strike out. Almost one-half of the children were judged to have problems related to eating and mealtimes, either not eating well or eating too much. Outside of mealtimes, they all placed objects in their mouth, and the majority had actually swallowed or consumed non-food items (including stones, paper, glue, and plastic) thereby causing a health and safety concern.

The issue of whether the previously mentioned behavior patterns are specifically related to AS or are found among individuals who are functioning at a similar developmental level but do not have the same underlying genetic abnormality could not be addressed by the within-syndrome approach that was used by the investigators. A study by Summers and Feldman (1999), however, was designed to determine whether AS is associated with a distinctive pattern of behavioral functioning. In order to do so, 27 children and young adults with AS (mean age of 9 years) were matched to individuals with developmental disability of mixed etiology on the basis of age, gender and level of intellectual functioning. The comparison groups came from two sources: (1) a behavior management service for children and young adults with developmental disabilities ("clinic group"); and (2) participants in an Ontario-wide survey of the prevalence of behavior problems among individuals with developmental disabilities ("community group"). A standardized rating scale (the Aberrant Behavior Checklist) (Aman & Singh, 1986) was completed by parents/caregivers and was used to gather information about maladaptive behavior patterns among the participants. The results of the study provided the first empirical evidence in support of a specific profile of behavior in individuals with AS, in that they scored significantly lower on measures of irritability and lethargy/social withdrawal than the two comparison groups. These findings are consistent with clinical observations of the happy demeanor and sociable disposition of individuals with AS.

Clarke and Marston (2000) also used the Aberrant Behavior Checklist to study behavioral functioning in a group of individuals with AS who were deletion positive. In this study, scores obtained by 61 individuals with AS who ranged in age from 6-21 years were compared to norms that were derived from a large sample of students with developmental disabilities who lived in community settings. The findings indicated that the AS group scored lower on measures of lethargy and inappropriate speech than the community comparison group. The effect of age on behavioral functioning was investigated by dividing the sample into groups of under 16 years and over 16 years. The only significant finding to emerge was a negative correlation between age and scores on a measure of hyperactivity and noncompliance, such that scores tended to decrease (indicating less severe problems) with increasing age. The Reiss Screen for Maladaptive Behavior (Reiss, 1988) was used to screen for signs of severe mental illness, which was not detected among any of the individuals who were assessed. Other problem or unusual behaviors that were reported by caregivers included a fascination with water or excessive water play, eating problems, sleep problems and mouthing or trying to eat non-food items.

Despite methodological differences among these studies, a fairly consistent picture emerges regarding the range of behavioral issues reported among individuals with AS. There is, however, more variation regarding the prevalence of different behaviors. The finding of a specific profile of behavioral functioning among individuals with AS is important from a clinical and therapeutic standpoint. Knowledge of developmental and behavioral issues that are likely to be associated with a diagnosis of AS may aid in the selection and timing of treatment approaches, provide prognostic information, and promote proactive planning efforts.

Intervention Studies

The majority of the literature to date has focused on the genetic, medical, and developmental aspects of AS. A small number of studies have reported the results of intervention efforts. These intervention studies will be presented briefly in this section.

Sleep Disturbance

Sleep disturbance is a very common occurrence among individuals with AS and may affect up to 90% of the population at some point in their lives (Clayton-Smith, 1993; Smith et al., 1996). A number of sleep-related problems have been reported, including problems initiating and maintaining sleep, early wakenings, high levels of nocturnal motor activity, and disruptive behavior during the night. The etiology of the sleep disturbance is unknown but may be related to abnormalities in brain development as well as the use of anti-convulsant medication that contains sodium valproate, a compound which acts to suppress blood melatonin levels (Zhdanova, Wurtman, & Wagstaff, 1999).

Summers et al. (1992) used a combined behavioral and pharmacological approach to treat a sleep-wake schedule disorder in a 9-year-old boy with AS. Before treatment, he slept an average of 1.9 hours during the night and 1.3 hours during the day. Treatment consisted of keeping him awake during the day whenever possible; restricting his access to fluids in the early evening to prevent him from wakening due to being wet; administering a small dose of a medication that induces drowsiness (diphenhydramine hydrochloride) an hour before bedtime; establishing a consistent bed time; and redirecting him back to bed if he got up during the night. Following the introduction of treatment (which was carried out initially in a hospital setting), the child's night sleep increased to an average of 8.3 hours and his day sleep was reduced to an average of .08 hours. Medication was discontinued subsequently and his night sleep decreased slightly while his day sleep was unaffected. His mother implemented the program once he returned home from hospital. The information she was able to collect indicated that his night and day sleep remained stable. Thus, behavioral methods alone were used to successfully maintain a stable sleep pattern at home once the medication was discontinued. Since the follow-up period was relatively short (45 days), however, it was not known whether the treatment gains were maintained long term.

Zhdanova et al. (1999) studied the effects of a low dose of melatonin on sleep in 13 children with AS who ranged in age from 2-10 years. Administration of the medication resulted in a more regular pattern of sleep onset and an increased total period of sleep in the majority of children studied. As well, lowered levels of nocturnal motor activity were found, reflecting an overall improvement in the children's nighttime sleep pattern (i.e., less interrupted sleep).

Due to what are likely pervasive effects of sleep disturbance on individuals with AS and their family members, it is likely that sleep-related issues will be the focus of ongoing research in the years to come.

Toileting

As mentioned earlier in the chapter (Table 3, Adaptive Functioning), there is evidence that many adolescents and adults with AS are able to achieve bladder and bowel control, primarily during the day. However, many individuals remain incontinent, an occurrence which has implications for their health and functional independence. Didden, Sikkema, Bosman, Duker, and Curfs (2001) modified an established toileting program in an attempt to train daytime continence in 6 children and adolescents with AS who ranged in age from 6-19 years. The intensive program (lasting an average of 6.5 hours/day) consisted of several elements: consumption of fluids every 30 minutes; conducting pant checks every 5 minutes and immediately reinforcing dry pants; providing toileting opportunities every 30 minutes; reinforcing successful eliminations in the toilet; and requiring individuals to change their clothing, clean the soiled area, and to sit on a chair without having access to toys when an accident occurred. The mean frequency of successful eliminations in the toilet went from 0.8 times per day before training to an average of 3.5 times per day after intensive training. Concurrently, the number of accidents declined from an average of 1.7 times per day before training to an average of 0.7 times per day after training. It took 17 days on average for individuals to reach a pre-determined criterion for success; the total time invested in training each individual ranged from 78-156 hours. It was encouraging to note that toileting successes were maintained at a 2.5 year follow-up.

Special Issues

This section will briefly touch upon issues that have not been covered elsewhere in the chapter.

Parent Support

Families of individuals with AS face a number of challenges. Some of these challenges are experienced by families of children with disabilities in general. Other challenges, however, may be specifically related to having a child with AS. In order to provide effective and timely supports and services, it is important for professionals to understand parents' issues. Van den Borne, van Hooren, van Gestel, Fryns, and Curfs (1999) surveyed parents about their response to having a child with AS and how they were able to cope with this (parents of children with Prader Willi syndrome were surveyed as well). Twenty-two families who had a young child with AS (mean age of 7 years) participated in the study. Most families indicated a strong need for information about the prospects for their child's development and education. They wanted to know more about the purpose of different treatments, including medication and physical and speech therapy. They wanted to learn about the best way to deal with their child and how to talk to family members and friends about the difficulties posed by their child's disability. Many parents indicated a need for information about how other parents coped with their child's disability and wondered how to connect with other AS parents. Many expressed fears about whether their child would receive sufficient care in the future and were concerned about the possibility of having to always depend on other people because of their child's disability. In terms of the emotional, physical and financial burdens posed by having a child with AS, many parents identified that they needed to spend much more time on their child's education; had the feeling that things didn't come as easily as they had before; had less time to attend to their job, household duties and leisure pursuits; and had increased special expenses. On a positive note, having a child with AS did not appear to have a detrimental effect on parents' self-esteem, as most identified that they were satisfied with themselves and had a positive self-attitude.

Safety Issues

Individuals with AS may be at particular risk for accidental injury or even death. Some of the factors that may have a bearing on this issue include their lack of awareness of potential hazards or dangers; characteristically high levels of activity, combined with a short attention span and impulsivity; and a tendency to engage in particular behaviors (e.g., mouthing or swallowing non-food items or involvement in water-related activities). As a result, constant and close supervision, along with hazard-proofing the environment, are required to maintain the safety of the individual with AS. A compelling reminder of the need for constant vigilance was provided by a report of drowning as an accidental cause of death in a 9-year-old boy with AS (Ishmael, Begleiter, & Butler, 2002). The child had managed to escape unnoticed into the backyard and was found floating in a shallow wading pool. There was the possibility that he had suffered a seizure while in the pool.

Future Directions for Intervention Research

Many exciting discoveries have been made into the underlying genetic causes of AS. Along with these discoveries comes the finding that AS is associated with a broader spectrum of clinical features and functional abilities than once thought. While research efforts to date have focused primarily on the genetic, medical and developmental aspects of AS, intervention studies are now starting to appear in the literature. Future directions for intervention research may include consideration of the following:

- ◆ gearing intervention toward teaching functional, adaptive skills in individuals with AS (e.g., communication, play, social, motor, self-care skills) and improving their "readiness to learn" skills (e.g., attention, imitation) as a way to promote greater competence and independence and ultimately a more positive quality of life. There is a vast literature, for instance, on using approaches that are based on applied behavior analysis to teach skills to individuals with severe and profound developmental disabilities to draw from in this regard.

- ◆ using a longitudinal approach and collecting standardized, quantifiable data to document developmental changes in individuals with AS and to evaluate the impact of different interventions (e.g., medical, behavioral, educational) on various indices of their functioning.

- ◆ using inter and multi-disciplinary approaches that incorporate contributions from different disciplines (e.g., neurology and various medical specialties; physical, speech and behavior therapy; psychology; special education) to provide services and supports to individuals with AS.

- ◆ empowering parents by providing them with useful and timely information about AS and related issues and helping them to become effective advocates for services and supports for their children.

Acknowledgments

The authors would like to thank the families who kindly permitted information about their sons and daughters to be used in the chapter and the service providers who provided additional information. Many thanks are also due to Charles A. Williams, M.D. for his helpful comments about the chapter.

Resources

Angelman Syndrome Foundation
414 Plaza Drive, Suite 209

Westmount, IL 60559
Phone: 800.IF.ANGEL or 630-734-9267
Fax: 630-655-0391
E-mail info@angelman.org
Web site: www.angelman.org

Canadian Angelman Syndrome Society
P.O. Box 37, Priddis, Alberta T0L 1W0
Phone: 403-931-2415
Fax: 403-931-4237
E-mail:info@angelmancanada.org
Web site: www.angelmancanada.org

References

Alvares, R. L. (2000). Survey of expressive communication skills in Angelman syndrome: An update. Paper presented at the 1st World Conference of the International Angelman Syndrome Organization, Tampere, Finland.

Alvares, R. L., & Downing, S. F. (1998). A survey of expressive communication skills in children with Angelman syndrome. *American Journal of Speech-Language Pathology, 7,* 14-24.

Aman, M. G., & Singh, N. N. (1986). *Aberrant Behavior Checklist: Manual.* E. Aurora, NY: Slosson Educational Publications Inc.

American Society of Human Genetics/American College of Medical Genetics Test and Technology Transfer Committee. (1996). Diagnostic testing for Prader-Willi and Angelman syndromes: Report of the ASHG/ACMG Test and Technology Transfer Committee. *American Journal of Human Genetics, 58,* 1085-1088.

Andersen, W. H., Rasmussen, R. K., & Stromme, P. (2001). Levels of cognitive and linguistic development in Angelman children: A study of 20 children. *Logopedics, Phoniatrics, Vocology, 26,* 2-9.

Angelman, H. (1965). 'Puppet' children: A report on three cases. *Developmental Medicine and Child Neurology, 7,* 681-688.

Beukelman, D. R., & Mirenda, P. (1992). *Augmentative and alternative communication. Management of severe communication disorders in children and adults.* Baltimore, MD: Paul H. Brookes.

Bottani, A., Robinson, W. P., DeLozier-Blanchet, D. D., Engel, E., Morris, M. A., Schmitt, B., et al. (1994). Angelman syndrome due to paternal uniparental disomy of chromosome 15: A milder phenotype? *American Journal of Medical Genetics, 51,* 35-40.

Buckley, R. H., Dinno, N., & Weber, P. (1998). Angelman syndrome: Are the estimates too low? *American Journal of Medical Genetics, 80,* 385-390.

Buntinx, I. M., Hennekam, R. C. M., Brouwer, O. F., Stroink, H., Beuten, J., Mangelschots, K., et al. (1995). Clinical profile of Angelman syndrome at different ages. *American Journal of Medical Genetics, 56*, 176-183.

Butler, M. G., & Palmer, C. G. (1983). Parental origin of chromosome 15 deletion in Prader-Willi syndrome (Letter). *Lancet, 1 (8336)*, 1285-1286.

Chan, C. T. J., Clayton-Smith, J., Cheng, X. J., Buxton, J., Webb, T., Pembrey, M. E., & Malcolm, S. (1993). Molecular mechanisms in Angelman syndrome: A survey of 93 patients. *Journal of Medical Genetics, 30*, 895-902.

Clarke, D. J., & Marston, G. (2000). Problem behaviors associated with 15q- Angelman syndrome. *American Journal on Mental Retardation, 105*, 25-31.

Clayton-Smith, J. (1993). Clinical research on Angelman syndrome in the United Kingdom: Observations on 82 affected individuals. *American Journal of Medical Genetics, 46*, 12-15.

Clayton-Smith, J. (1995). On the prevalence of Angelman syndrome. *American Journal of Medical Genetics, 59*, 403-404.

Clayton-Smith, J. (2001). Angelman syndrome: Evolution of the phenotype in adolescents and adults. *Developmental Medicine and Child Neurology, 43*, 476-480.

Clayton-Smith, J., & Pembrey, M.E. (1992). Angelman syndrome. *Journal of Medical Genetics, 29*, 412-415.

Didden, R., Sikkema, S. P. E., Bosman, I. T. M., Duker, P. C., & Curfs, L. M. G. (2001). Use of a modified Azrin-Foxx toilet training procedure with individuals with Angelman syndrome. *Journal of Applied Research in Intellectual Disabilities, 14*, 64-70.

Driscoll, D. J. (1994). Genomic imprinting in humans. *Molecular Genetics Medicine, 4*, 37-77.

Fisher, J. A., Burn, J., Alexander, F. W., & Gardner-Medwin, D. (1987). Angelman (happy puppet) syndrome in a girl and her brother. *Journal of Medical Genetics, 24*, 294-298.

Fryburg, J. S., Breg, W. R., & Lindgren, V. (1991). Diagnosis of Angelman syndrome in infants. *American Journal of Medical Genetics, 38*, 58-64.

Ginsburg, H., & Opper, S. (1979). *Piaget's theory of intellectual development (2nd Edition)*. Englewood Cliffs, N.J: Prentice-Hall, Inc.

Hersh, J. H., Bloom, A. S., Zimmerman, A. W., Dinno, N. D., Greenstein, R. M., Weisskopf, B., et al. (1981). Behavioral correlates in the happy puppet syndrome: A characteristic profile? *Developmental Medicine and Child Neurology, 23*, 792-800.

Ishmael, H. A., Begleiter, M. L., & Butler, M. G. (2002). Drowning as a cause of death in Angelman syndrome. *American Journal on Mental Retardation, 107*, 69-70.

Jacobsen, J., King, B. H., Leventhal, B. L., Christian, S. L., Ledbetter, D. H., & Cook, E. H. (1998). Molecular screening for proximal 15q abnormalities in a mentally retarded population. *Journal of Medical Genetics, 35,* 534-538.

Jiang, Y. H., Lev-Lehman, E., Bressler, J., Tsai, T. F., & Beaudet, A. (1999). Genetics of Angelman syndrome. *American Journal of Human Genetics, 65,* 1-6.

Jolleff, N., & Ryan, M. M. (1993). Communication development in Angelman's syndrome. *Archives of Disease in Childhood, 69,* 148-150.

Kaplan, L. C., Wharton, R., Elias, E., Mandell, F., Donlon, T., & Latt, S.A. (1987). Clinical heterogeneity associated with deletions in the long arm of chromosome 15: Report of 3 new cases and their possible genetic significance. *American Journal of Medical Genetics, 28,* 45-53.

Kishino, T., Lalande, M., & Wagstaff, J. (1997). UBE3A/E6-AP mutations cause Angelman syndrome. *Nature Genetics, 15,* 70-73.

Knoll, J. H. M., Nicholls, R. D., Magenis, R. E., Graham, J. M., Lalande, M., & Latt, S. A. (1989). Angelman and Prader-Willi sydromes share a common chromosome 15 deletion but differ in the parental origin of the deletion. *American Journal of Medical Genetics, 32,* 285-290.

Laan, L. A. E. M., Th. den Boer, A., Hennekam, R. C. M., Renier, W. O., & Brouwer, O. F. (1996). Angelman syndrome in adulthood. *American Journal of Medical Genetics, 66,* 356-360.

Lombroso, P. J. (2000). Genetics of childhood disorders: XVI. Angelman syndrome: A failure to process. *Journal of the American Academy of Child and Adolescent Psychiatry, 39,* 931-933.

Lossie, A. C., & Driscoll, D. J. (1999). Transmission of Angelman syndrome by an affected mother. *Genetics in Medicine, 1,* 262-266.

Magenis, R. E., Brown, M. G., Lacy, D. A., Budden, S., & LaFranchi. S. (1987). Is Angelman syndrome an alternate result of del(15)(q11q13)? *American Journal of Medical Genetics, 28,* 829-838.

Malcolm, S., Clayton-Smith, J., Nichols, M., Robb, S., Webb, T., Armour, J. A. L., et al. (1991). Uniparental paternal disomy in Angelman's syndrome. *Lancet, 337,* 694-697.

Moncla, A., Malzac, P., Livet, M. O., Voelckel, M. A., Mancini, J., Delaroziere, J. C., et al. (1999a). Angelman syndrome resulting from UBE3A mutations in 14 patients from eight families: Clinical manifestations and genetic counselling. *Journal of Medical Genetics, 36,* 554-560.

Moncla, A., Malzac, P., Voelckel, M. A., Auquier, P., Girardot, L., Mattei, M. G., et al. (1999b). Phenotype-genotype correlation in 20 deletion and 20 non-deletion Angelman syndrome patients. *European Journal of Human Genetics, 7,* 131-139.

Oliver, C., Demetriades, L., & Hall, S. (2002). Effects of environmental events on smiling and laughing behavior in Angelman syndrome. *American Journal on Mental Retardation, 107,* 194-200.

Penner, K. A., Johnston, J., Faircloth, B. H., Irish, P., & Williams, C. A. (1993). Communication, cognition and social interaction in the Angelman syndrome. *American Journal of Medical Genetics, 46,* 34-39.

Reiss, S. (1988). *Reiss Screen for Maladaptive Behavior test manual.* Worthington, OH: IDS.

Rougeulle, C., Glatt, H., & Lalande, M. (1997). The Angelman syndrome candidate gene, UBE3A/E6-AP, is imprinted in brain. *Nature Genetics, 17,* 14-15.

Sandanam, T., Beange, H., Robson, L., Woolnough, H., Buchholz, T., & Smith, A. (1997). Manifestations in institutionalized adults with Angelman syndrome due to deletion. *American Journal of Medical Genetics, 70,* 415-420.

Smith, A., Wiles, A., Haan, E., McGill, J., Wallace, G., Dixon, J., et al. (1996). Clinical features in 27 patients with Angelman syndrome resulting from DNA deletion. *Journal of Medical Genetics, 33,* 107-112.

Steffenburg, S., Gillberg, C. L., Steffenburg, U., & Kyllerman, M. (1996). Autism in Angelman syndrome: A population-based study. *Pediatric Neurology, 14,* 131-136.

Summers, J. A., Allison, D. B., Lynch, P. S., & Sandler, L. (1995). Behaviour problems in Angelman syndrome. *Journal of Intellectual Disability Research, 39,* 97-106.

Summers, J. A., & Feldman, M. A. (1999). Distinctive pattern of behavioral functioning in Angelman syndrome. *American Journal on Mental Retardation, 104,* 376-384.

Summers, J. A., Lynch, P. S., Harris, J. C., Burke, J. C., Allison, D. B., & Sandler, L. (1992). A combined behavioral/pharmacological treatment of sleep-wake schedule disorder in Angelman syndrome. *Journal of Developmental and Behavioral Pediatrics, 13,* 284-287.

Van den Borne, H. W., van Hooren, R. H., van Gestel, M., Fryns, J. P., & Curfs, L. M. G. (1999). Psychosocial problems, coping strategies, and the need for information of parents of children with Prader-Willi syndrome and Angelman syndrome. *Patient Education and Counselling, 38,* 205-216.

Van Lierde, A., Atza, M. G., Giardino, D., & Viani, F. (1990). Angelman's syndrome in the first year of life. *Developmental Medicine and Child Neurology, 32,* 1011-1016.

Wilcox, D. (1991). Heather's story: The long road for a family in search of a diagnosis. *Exceptional Parent, 21,* 92-94.

Willems, P. J., Dijkstra, I., Brouwer, O. F., & Smit, G. P. A. (1987). Recurrence risk in the Angelman ("happy puppet") syndrome. *American Journal of Medical Genetics, 27,* 773-780.

Williams, C. A., Angelman, H., Clayton-Smith, J., Driscoll, D. J., Hendrickson, J. E., Knoll, J. H. M., et al. (1995a). Angelman syndrome: Consensus for diagnostic criteria. *American Journal of Medical Genetics, 56*, 237-238.

Williams, C. A., Lossie, A., & Driscoll, D. (2001). Angelman syndrome: Mimicking conditions and phenotypes. *American Journal of Medical Genetics, 101*, 59-64.

Williams, C. A., Zori, R. T., Hendrickson, J., Stalker, H., Marum, T., Whidden, E., et al. (1995b). Angelman syndrome. *Current Problems in Pediatrics, 25*, 216-231.

Williams, C. A., Zori, R. T., Stone, J. W., Gray, B. A., Cantu, E. S., & Ostrer, H. (1990). Maternal origin of 15q11-13 deletions in Angelman syndrome suggests a role for genomic imprinting. *American Journal of Medical Genetics, 35*, 350-353.

Yamada, K. A., & Volpe, J. J. (1990). Angelman's syndrome in infancy. *Developmental Medicine and Child Neurology, 32*, 1005-1010.

Yussen, S. R., & Santrock, J.W. (1982). *Child development: An introduction (2nd Ed.).* Dubuque, IA: Wm. Brown Company.

Zhdanova, I. V., Wurtman, R. J., & Wagstaff, J. (1999). Effects of a low dose of melatonin on sleep in children with Angelman syndrome. *Journal of Pediatric Endocrinology and Metabolism, 12*, 57-67.

Zori, R. T., Hendrickson, J., Woolven, S., Whidden, E. M., Gray, B. & Williams, C. A. (1992). Angelman syndrome: Clinical profile. *Journal of Child Neurology, 7*, 270-278.

CHAPTER 9

Tourette Syndrome

Robert King, Garry Fay, & Heather Prescott

Introduction

Although the first case report of Tourette syndrome (TS) was written in 1663 by Drage (Lees, Robertson, Trimble, & Murray, 1984), Georges Gilles de la Tourette, in citing nine cases in 1885, was the first to comprehensively describe the triad of (1) multiple tics, (2) involuntary movements and (3) echolalia. TS is now known to be a neurochemical disorder characterized by frequent motor and phonic tics, with a childhood onset and a fluctuating course, a duration of greater than one year and associated distress or significant impairment in social, occupational or other important areas of functioning (DSM-IV) (American Psychiatric Association, 1994).

Little attention was paid to this disorder for many years subsequent to this description, in both individuals with and without developmental disabilities (DD). The first case series describing TS in individuals with DD (Golden & Greenhill, 1981) documented TS in children with borderline to severe degrees of cognitive impairment and favorable results (at the expense of dyskinetic adverse effects) in response to the medication Haloperidol. These authors noted that prior to the diagnosis of TS, tics in these children had been attributed to psychotic disorders or anxiety. They also

189

insightfully speculated that the same organic insults contributing to DD in these children could potentially be implicated in the etiology of their TS.

More recently, significant advances have occurred in the understanding of the etiology and treatment of TS and its comorbid or co-occurring conditions. In addition, the natural history of TS and its impact upon self-esteem, family and peer relationships, vocational and educational performance, and overall quality of life are now well described.

This chapter will review these advances, acknowledging that little of this research has involved individuals with DD and TS. Whenever possible, however, the implications of this work in supporting individuals with TS and DD will be highlighted. Particular attention will be paid to (1) diagnostic and systemic issues that have acted as historical barriers to an accurate determination of the prevalence of TS in individuals with DD, (2) a description of the emerging potential relationship between TS and pervasive developmental disorders (PDD), and (3) the art of providing safe and efficacious pharmacological, behavioral and habilitative support to individuals with TS/DD and associated complex comorbid conditions.

Epidemiology

The accepted prevalence of TS is 1-8/1,000 in males and 0.1-4/1,000 in females (Peterson, 1996). Increasingly it is recognized that many mild cases of TS do not come to clinical attention and that these rates likely underestimate the true prevalence. No comprehensive attempt has been made to establish the prevalence of TS in community-based samples of individuals with DD. Eapen, Robertson, Zeitlin, and Kurlan (1997) compared the prevalence of tic disorders in children from a residential school for individuals with emotional and behavioral difficulties, a residential school for individuals with learning disabilities and a group of children identified as having academic or behavioral problems. Tics were identified in 65%, 29% and 6% of representative samples of each of these groups. Kurlan, Whitmore, Irvine, McDermott, Como (1994) noted a prevalence of tics in 26% of special education students vs. 6% of regular classroom students. Comings, Himes, and Comings (1990), in a study of a single California school district, estimated that 20% of children in special education have a tic disorder.

In a tertiary care clinical setting, Myers and Pueschel (1995) noted a prevalence of TS of 1.2% in 425 individuals with Down syndrome. They noted that case reports have documented the co-occurrence of TS and many other chromosomal abnormalities, including XYY, XXY, 9p monomy, fragile X syndrome and 9p mosaicism.

In addition, Burd, Fisher, Kerbeshian, and Arnold (1987) reported a 20% prevalence (12/59) of TS in a group of individuals with PDD. Case reports of individuals with comorbid TS and Asperger's syndrome have also been documented.

There remains a critical need for epidemiological research to establish the true prevalence in individuals with DD, particularly to identify possible differences amongst groups of individuals with known etiologies for their disabilities. An improved understanding of the assumed heterogeneous etiology of TS and syndrome-specific treatment implications could theoretically arise from such research.

Etiology

Multiple lines of inquiry regarding the etiology of TS are currently being investigated and are discussed below.

Genetic Etiologies

Genetic studies to date of TS are most consistent with a model of autosomal dominant inheritance with incomplete penetrance (50% of the children of an identified parent with TS are at risk, with some unexplained variability). An international genetic research consortium appears close to identifying the TS gene currently (Walkup, 1999). Twin studies (Price, Kidd, Cohen, Pauls, & Leckman, 1985) have identified a 53% concordance rate in monozygotic twins vs. an 8% concordance rate in dizygotic twins. This difference suggests that there are both genetic and non-genetic factors contributing to the etiology of TS. Leckman, Price, Walkup, Ort, Pauls, and Cohen (1987) have noted that amongst discordant monozygotic twins, the unaffected twin has a higher birth weight, emphasizing the role of non-genetic factors in determining penetrance (including placental function, intrauterine crowding, pre and perinatal hypoxia and ischemic insults). Interestingly, these factors are also capable of producing more generalized cognitive impairments, possibly linking the co-occurrence of DD and TS in some individuals. *Family studies* have demonstrated a tenfold increased risk of TS in parents or siblings of affected individuals. No genetic studies have been completed in individuals with TS and DD. In a case review of seven children with DD and TS, Goldman (1988) noted that negative family histories of TS in some children were confounded by the attribution of tics in some parents, to anxiety associated with parenting a child with DD. There is no scientific reason to believe that the genetic findings to date in individuals with TS will not hold for individuals with TS and DD.

Neurobiological and Neuroanatomic Etiologies

Hypotheses regarding abnormalities of the neurochemical dopamine in the basal ganglia and the prefrontal cortical areas of the brain are supported by therapeutic responses (tic suppression) to medications which antagonize dopamine and tic exacerbation by stimulant medication (Lowe, Cohen, Detlor, Kremenitzer, & Shaywitz, 1982). Magnetic resonance imaging (MRI) studies have demonstrated a loss of the usual left-right asymmetry of the putamen in the basal ganglia, the proposed neurobiological substrate of TS. Dr. Daniel Weinberger as quoted in *The New York Times* (Blakeslee, 1996), observed that more severely affected monozygotic twins have highly sensitive D_2 (dopamine) receptors on the head of the caudate nucleus (also a part of the basal ganglia) proposing a *faulty neurological braking system model of TS*. This model suggests that the caudate nucleus sensitivity to dopamine impairs the caudate's usual function of selectively stopping movements. As a result, tics are allowed to be expressed as fragments of movements or thoughts split off from integrated movements.

Neuroimaging and neurobiological studies also suggest basal ganglia dysfunction in TS. Specific circuits involved in mediating behavioral initiation, monitoring, and inhibition, linking the cerebral cortex, the thalamus, and the basal ganglia, are thought to be malfunctional in TS.

Autoimmune/Infectious Etiologies

Observations of tics and compulsive behavior in children with Sydenham's chorea, a neurological sequelae of rheumatic fever, have lead Swedo et al. (1997) and others to propose a *molecular mimicry model of TS.* A subset of individuals with TS have been discovered to have *pediatric autoimmune neuropsychiatric disorders associated with streptococcal infection (PANDAS).* Clinical presentations of this disorder are characterized by symptom exacerbations with abrupt onsets which are temporally related to group A B(beta)-hemolytic streptococcal infections. Antibodies against this bacteria have been demonstrated to cross-react with neural antibodies in the basal ganglia resulting in inflammation (Perlmutter et al., 1999). This work is yet to be extended to individuals with TS and DD.

The Etiological Relationship Between Autism and TS

In reviewing sixteen individuals with PD and TS, Comings and Comings (1991) proposed a genetic relationship between these two disorders. Sverd (1991) noted various manifestations of the TS gene in family members of ten individuals studied with autism and TS, suggesting again support for the hypothesis that TS contributes to the etiological heterogeneity of autism. Both authors have speculated that autism and TS may be a more severe expression of the homozygotic form of the TS gene. Kerbeshian and Burd (1986) have described the occurrence of TS, autism, fragile X syndrome and moderate mental retardation (MR) in an individual. Clinical similarities between TS and autism are highlighted below.

Similarities Between Autism and TS

- ♦ Delays in speech development
- ♦ Onset in childhood
- ♦ A male predominance
- ♦ Ritualistic (or compulsive) behavior
- ♦ Adverse reactions to minor environmental change
- ♦ The significant smelling of objects

MRI imaging of seven children with TS and Asperger's syndrome has demonstrated structural brain abnormalities not seen in a controlled group of children with TS alone (Berthier, Bayes, & Tolosa, 1993).

Diagnostic and Assessment Issues

Table 1. DSM-IV Criteria for Tourette's Disorder

a) Both multiple motor or one or more vocal tics have been present at some time during the illness, although not necessarily concurrently (a tic is a sudden, rapid, recurrent, non-rhythmic stereotyped motor movement or vocalization).

b) The tics occur many times a day (usually in bouts), nearly every day or intermittently throughout a period of more than one year and during this period, there was never a tic-free period of more than three consecutive months.

c) The disturbance causes marked distress or significant impairment in social, occupational, or other important areas of functioning.

d) The onset is before age 18 years.

e) The disturbance is not due to the direct physiological effects of a substance (for example, stimulants) or a general medical condition (for example, Huntington's disease or post-viral encephalitis).

Tics are classified according to the involvement of a single muscle (*simple*) or a group of muscles (*complex*), as well as being either **motor** or **phonic** phenomena. Distinguishing features of tics are enumerated in Table 2.

Table 2. Distinguishing Features of Tics

1. Abrupt onset
2. Preceded by sensory phenomena (premonitory urges)
3. Involuntary but temporarily suppressible
4. Decreased with distraction
5. Increased with stress, fatigue, and excitement
6. Are multiform and may involve any muscle in the body
7. Intensity and frequency may fluctuate spontaneously
8. Can be present during sleep

The *natural history* of TS in individuals without DD is graphically depicted in Graph 1 and is characterized by an early childhood onset, prepubertal exacerbations, postpubertal attenuation concluding with degrees of stabilization in adulthood.

Graph 1. Natural History of TS

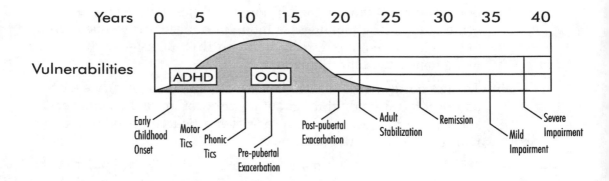

1. **An early childhood onset** - 50% of children with TS have a preceding history of an attention deficit disorder with hyperactivity (ADHD). The average age of motor tic onset is 7 years. This is followed by an average age of phonic tic onset of 9 years. Initial tics frequently include forcible eye blinking, facial grimacing, head jerking, licking of lips with a progression of tics from head to neck to upper extremities to lower extremities over time.

2. **A prepubertal exacerbation** - After approximately age 10-11, individuals with TS are able to describe the awareness of a *premonitory urge* (a vague discomfort or urge to move in the region where the tic may occur) (Peterson, 1996). Eliciting this information historically can assist the clinician in distinguishing a complex motor tic from a compulsion, which is in contrast typically preceded by anxiety and the occurrence of an obsession. Approximately 50% of children with TS beginning at age 10-11 ultimately develop comorbid obsessive compulsive disorder (OCD). The DSM-IV criteria for OCD are as follows:

   1. **Compulsions:**
      a. Repetitive behaviors (example, hand washing, ordering, checking) or mental acts (praying, counting, repeating words silently) that the person feels driven to perform in response to an obsession or according to rules that must be rigidly applied.
      b. The behaviors or mental acts are aimed at preventing or reducing distress or preventing some dreaded event or situation; however, these behaviors or mental acts either are not connected in a realistic way with what they are designed to neutralize or prevent or are clearly excessive.

   2. **Obsessions:**
      a. Recurrent or persistent thoughts, impulses, or images that are experienced, at some time during the disturbance, as intru-

sive and inappropriate and that cause marked anxiety or distress.

b. The thoughts, impulses or images are not simply excessive worries about real life problems.

c. The person attempts to ignore or suppress such thoughts, impulses or images or to neutralize them with some thought or action.

d. The person recognizes that the obsessional thoughts, impulses „or images are a product of his or her own mind (not imposed from without as in thought insertion).

3. **Postpubertal attenuation** of tic severity and frequency

4. **Adult stabilization:**
   - ◆ One third will experience remission
   - ◆ One third will experience milder tics than in childhood
   - ◆ One third will continue to have severe tics and functional impairment (Peterson and Cohen, 1998)

The natural history of TS in individuals with DD is uncharted. In Golden and Greenhill's 1981 case series, a childhood onset of tics was noted in all six cases. Reid (1984) described the late adolescent onset of tics in a 33-year-old female with mild MR and a comorbid psychotic disorder and seizure disorder. The onset of phonic tics at age 30, although felt to be consistent with the natural history of TS by Reid at the time of the report's writing, is now known to be atypical, suggesting possible other etiologies. Goldman (1988) described seven children with varying degrees of DD (mild to profound), including two with autistic disorders. Each presented with a severe behavioral disorder, resulting in Goldman's recommendation that "particular care should be taken to observe for TS embedded in the early and intractable behavior syndrome of hyperactivity, agitation, aggressivity and non-compliance". It seems reasonable to anticipate similar ages of tic onset in individuals with TS based upon these reports. In working with an adult population with DD and TS, the authors have observed that retrospective reviews of previous assessments often confirm a focus on challenging behaviors (aggression, sleep disturbance or self-injury). Not uncommonly, this creates a barrier to an accurate retrospective estimation of the chronology of tic and comorbid conditions.

Cross-sectionally, in individuals with DD and suspected TS, tic-like movement disorders must be distinguished from a variety of other conditions. These are listed in Table 3.

Table 3. Differential Diagnosis of Tics

1. **Tardive Dyskinesia** - involuntary, repetitive, less rhythmic, typically orofacial movements arising as an adverse effect of exposure to antipsychotic medication.

2. **Stereopyties** - rhythmic, usually bilateral, more prolonged whole body movements (body rocking, arm flapping) or object manipulations (string twirling) with a less rapid onset which can be temporarily suppressed. The distinction between stereopyties and complex motor tics can be particularly challenging in individuals with PDD.

3. **Compulsions** - (see previous definition). In individuals with TS and comorbid OCD, compulsions can be particularly difficult to distinguish from complex motor tics.

4. **Seizure Disorders** (especially movements associated with partial complex or frontal lobe seizures).

5. **Medication-induced Tics** (including Dilantin, Phenobarbital, Carbamazepine and Lamotrigine).

6. **Huntington's Disease**

7. **Encephalitis**

8. **Neuroacanthocytosis** (orofacial dyskinesias, lip and tongue biting and acanthocytes in red blood cells).

As indicated, the natural history of TS includes a strong link with a number of comorbid conditions. These are listed in Table 4.

Table 4. Comorbid Conditions in TS

1. Attention Deficit Hyperactive Disorder

2. Obssessive Compulsive Disorder

3. Anxiety Disorders

4. Affective Disorders

5. Learning Disabilities

6. Oppositional Defiant Disorder

Self-injurious behavior (SIB) is common in individuals with TS. In reviewing ninety individuals with TS, Robertson, Trimble, and Lees (1989) reported a 33% incident of SIB, the topography of which resembled SIB seen in individuals with severe DD, despite the fact that these individuals were of average intelligence. King (1999) has reported positive therapeutic outcomes in individuals with TS and DD based on the formulations that presenting SIB may represent either complex motor tics, or compulsions in the context of comorbid OCD.

Neuropsychological Findings

Neuropsychological studies in individuals with TS have focused on:

1. General intellectual ability.

2. Identifying specific learning disabilities. A 20% prevalence of math and written language disabilities is the most consistent finding (Yeates & Bornstein, 1996).

3. Documentation of specific neuropsychological deficits. Visual motor deficits on copying tasks are a consistent finding. Visual motor integration deficits are also, however, commonly documented in ADHD. Fine motor skill deficits (poor handwriting) are often noted. There is less compelling evidence for syndrome-specific spatial perceptual deficits.

Deficits of executive functioning (mental tracking, sustained attention, working memory, goal-directed behavior, impulse control, self-regulation, planning and sequencing, organizational skills and mental flexibility) have been commonly noted; however, these deficits are also again common in ADHD and OCD and some studies have suffered from failure to control for the presence of these comorbid conditions in test subjects. Neuropsychological study results have also been confounded by ascertainment bias (studying complex or severely effected clinic referred individuals), the effects of prescribed medication, the effect on mental functioning of active tic suppression, and the natural waxing and waning history of the disorder (Como, 1999).

No specific neuropsychological reports have been published involving individuals with TS and DD. Case reports have, however, clearly demonstrated TS in individuals with all degrees of DD. Ozonoff, Strayer, McMahon, and Filloux (1994) have suggested that executive function deficits may be responsible for the rigidity, perseverativeness, narrow focus on details and deficient ability to inhibit familiar or over-learned responses in PDD. These authors paralleled this formulation with the hypothesis that a similar executive and prefrontal cortex dysfunction in TS may result in a failure of a motor inhibitory system resulting in tics. Again, a link is suggested between TS and PDD by these authors.

Support Approaches

Given the challenges inherent in establishing a diagnosis of TS and its comorbid conditions in individuals with DD, support approaches must be individualized. Individualized support is premised on:

1. Knowledge of the degree of functional impairment in various domains of the individual's life associated with tic expression.

2. An awareness of the developmental context in which tics are occurring, particularly with respect to impact on peer relationships, family relationships, and self-esteem.

3. Knowledge regarding current and potential future impairment associated with comorbid conditions.

4. An understanding of available internal and external sources of support and capacity for coping (Peterson & Cohen, 1998).

Regardless of modality, support approaches should optimally be offered by a multidisciplinary team capable of objectively monitoring support and treatment outcomes.

Psychoeducation to clients, families, and caregivers has been identified as being the single most important treatment modality available. Critical information in this context includes:

1. The fact that tic severity by itself is a poor predictor of long-term overall prognosis. Quality of socialization (and intelligence in a non-disabled population) are best predictors of overall prognosis.

2. Significant impairment arising from comorbid conditions may be missed by an over-emphasis on tic suppression.

3. Knowledge of the natural history of TS (particularly the post-adolescent attenuation of tics) may inform decisions regarding potential deferment of pharmacological support and sustain hope regarding prognosis.

4. The impact of tic severity on self-esteem in TS is correlated with developmental stage (likely greatest in adolescence). This issue is often not considered in supporting individuals with DD and TS. A poor self-image in the context of moderate to severe cognitive impairment may be unrecognized as an antecedent to voluntary challenging behavior or as a risk factor for illnesses such as major depression.

5. Assisting caregivers in understanding that tics both wax and wane in severity and are involuntary, but temporarily suppressible. This knowledge assists in refuting beliefs that tics (especially complex motor tics and complex phonic tics), although potentially disruptive in classroom, life skills, recreational and vocational settings, are not under voluntary control; and should therefore not be the subject of punishment paradigms.

6. An emphasis on developing hypotheses regarding the etiology of aggression and self-injury as potential complex motor tics or compulsions or expressions of ADHD associated impulsivity, to allow rational pharmacological interventions. As illustrated in Table 5, support approaches to TS are multifaceted.

Table 5. Support Approaches to TS

1. Psychoeducation/psychotherapy
2. Pharmacotherapy
3. Immunotherapy
4. Behavior therapy
5. Educational, vocational, and habilitative supports

Pharmacotherapy

Tic suppression should be directed to improving quality of life through (1) improving self-esteem, (2) improving acceptance in interpersonal relationships and community integration, (3) decreasing distractibility, (4) reducing energy demands required to suppress tics, and (5) reducing tic interference with motor acts and speech (Peterson & Cohen, 1998). Tic suppressing pharmacological agents are illustrated in Table 6.

Multiple studies have demonstrated that low-dose risperidone is well tolerated in individuals with TS and DD/PDD in a variety of circumstances. King (1999) demonstrated its utility in three individuals with TS and DD as a tic suppressing agent, with additional improvement noted in aggression and oppositional behavior. As a 5-HT$_2$ antagonist, risperidone has been reported as having the potential to both augment anticompulsive agents in treating comorbid OCD (McDougle, Fleischmann, Epperson, Wasylink, Leckman, & Price, 1995) and exacerbating compulsions (Remington & Adams, 1994). Similar observations have been made with olanzapine (Mottard & De La Sablonniere, 1999) and clozapine (Patil, 1992).

The establishment of baseline parameters of expressed tics, as well as the signs and symptoms of comorbid conditions through operationally defining symptoms and choosing appropriate monitoring systems, is therefore critical to make global assessments of the merits of atypical antipsychotic agents. Clonidine is also an attractive alternative in a population of individuals with DD and TS, particularly if comorbid ADHD signs and symptoms of irritability, oppositional behavior, and a sleep disturbance are prominent.

Table 6. Pharmacological Management of Tics in Individuals With Developmental Disabilities

Drug	Dose Range	Expected Outcome	Common Adverse Effects
Adrenergic Agonists			
Clonidine	0.1 – 0.6 mg od (tid – qid)	tic suppression in 25 –50 % motor tics > phonic tics,improved sleep,improved attention and distractibility, decreased oppositional behavior	sedation, decreased blood pressure, dry mouth, irritability
Guanfacine	1-4 mg (bid – tid)	little experience in individuals with developmental disabilities	less sedation than clonidine
Dopamine Antagonists			
Haloperidol	1–3 mg (od – bid)	tic suppression in 70 – 80 %	67-89% experience intolerable side effects, acute dystonia, Parkinsonism, akathesia, sedation, sexual dysfunction, anti-cholinergic effects, tardive dyskinesia
Pimozide	1–4 mg (od – bid)	tic suppression in 70 –80 %	less sedation, prolonged QT intervals – arrhythmia
Atypical Anti-Psychotics			
Risperidone	1–6 mg (bid – tid)	tic suppression, decease in oppositional behavior	decreased risk of neurological adverse effects with an increasing dose, tardive dyskinesia, weight gain, hyperprolactinemia, sedation
Clozapine	300-600 mg (bid)	ineffective in single double blind study (Caine, Polinsky, Kartzinel, & Ebert, 1979) two case reports positive response tardive tourette's	agranulocytosis, hypersalivation, weight gain, and tachycardia
Olanzapine	5-20 mg (od)	effect on tardive dyskinesia in TS, 2 recent double-blind studies with positive results (Serrano & Pena, 1999; Stamenkovic, Willinger, & Kasper, 1999).	weight gain, sedation, no hyperprolactinemia, sexual dysfunction

Behavior Therapy

No large studies of the benefits of behavior therapy in individuals with TS and DD have been conducted. Zarkowska, Crawley; and Locke (1989) published a single case report of an attempt to treat a 13-year-old female with severe DD and TS with cue-controlled relaxation techniques. Tic frequency diminished during relaxation sessions, but these results could not be generalized outside of these sessions.

The following approaches have produced inconsistent results:

1. *Massed practice* - The deliberate performance of a tic, followed by a rest period, intended to produce reciprocal inhibition.
2. *Progressive muscle relaxation* - This procedure may non-specifically be helpful in individuals prone to exacerbations of tics induced by stress, and as a component of an anger management approach. Mental imagery has also been found to foster an improved sense of self-control in individuals with TS.
3. *Self-monitoring*
4. *Habit reversal* - The identification of a competing response for a targeted tic. Trials are currently under way investigating this promising approach (Como, 1999).

Impulsivity arising from comorbid ADHD and TS associated oppositional behavior may also benefit from:

1. Firm, consistent limit setting.
2. The use of planned withdrawal or access to a private area in a school or vocational setting to (a) decrease sensory and affective stimulation, and (b) allow the expression of tics without fear of censure or peer judgement.
3. Contingency rewards.

Immunotherapy

Early trials involving plasmarpheresis and intravenous gamma globulin treatment of children identified with PANDAS have shown promising results (Perlmutter et al., 1999). In addition, several studies have identified a B lymphocyte antigen, D8/17 in children with TS and childhood onset OCD, which may serve as a marker of susceptibility for these illnesses in genetically vulnerable sub-groups of children (Murphy et al., 1997; Swedo et al., 1997). Currently, multicentre longitudinal research trials are under way to strengthen these findings. Until further conclusions are drawn, the routine use of plasmapheresis, intravenous gamma globulin or penicillin prophylaxis in PANDAS identified children is not currently recommended.

Educational, Vocational and Habilitative Supports

Classroom support techniques include:

1. Educating peers.
2. Creating a quiet, separate space for test completion.
3. Asking the teacher to act as a role model, accepting tics with tolerance and patience.
4. Testing by modalities other than timed written examinations.
5. Assigning tasks one by one, rather than as a sequence.
6. Being aware of classroom and teaching modifications, addressing functional learning impairments caused by comorbid disorders.
7. Fostering self-worth.
8. Avoiding power struggles regarding "is this behavior a tic or not?" (for example, spitting may be a complex motor tic or a voluntary display of oppositional behavior - approaching this behavior as an unacceptable behavior

within the classroom while allowing free access to bathrooms, towels, quick exits from the classroom or other alternative solutions eliminates the need to attempt to make this distinction).

With modification, many of these principles are equally applicable to supporting individuals with DD and TS in recreational, pre-vocational, and vocational settings. Educating employers regarding the involuntary nature of tics is particularly important in establishing an atmosphere of acceptance in the workplace. Questions often arise regarding safety issues correlated with the expression of a motor tic while engaging in motor acts (for example, operating machinery or driving). For the vast majority of individuals with mild to moderate TS, the ability to temporarily suppress tics or develop compensatory strategies during their expression is adequate to ensure safety. In some situations, environmental modifications to the workplace or revision of job specification may be of benefit, as guided by an occupational therapy assessment.

Conclusions

Although the prevalence of TS in individuals with DD remains unknown, case series confirm the presence of this disorder in individuals with all degrees of cognitive impairment. Research confirming the heterogeneous etiology of TS parallels the heterogeneity of etiologies leading to DD, particularly in individuals with severe to profound degrees of cognitive impairment. Genetic and immunological theories of etiology of TS may in particular lead to promising new treatments of this disorder in the future.

The diagnosis of TS in individuals with DD remains challenging in a population in which a variety of other abnormal motor movements are over-represented and must be differentiated from tics. Knowledge of the natural history of TS and its comorbid conditions can assist clinicians in supporting or refuting the diagnosis of TS.

The establishment of the diagnosis of TS can lead to formulations regarding underlying etiologies of SIB, aggression, sleep disturbances, and over-activity; leading to rational treatment recommendations. In individuals with no verbal expressive skills, the inability to articulate the experience of premonitory urges or obsessions challenges the clinician in distinguishing between compulsions and complex motor tics as components, particularly of the presentation of SIB or aggression. In this context, it is critical for a multidisciplinary team to objectively monitor parameters of these target behaviors over time to judge their response to empirical treatment recommendations. Psychoeducation and pharmacotherapy remain the mainstays of treatment of tics and comorbid conditions of TS. Informed decision making regarding treatment recommendations is critically dependent upon the knowledge of the natural history of this disorder and its impact upon multiple aspects of the individual's quality of life. Educating family members, peers and caregivers regarding this disorder enhances the individual's coping capacities and resilience to the potential negative impact of this disorder on self-image and self-worth.

Continued documentation of the application of knowledge acquired from research involving individuals with TS but without DD, to individuals with DD and TS, will strengthen our support efforts for these individuals. Indeed, research specific to individuals with TS and DD would undoubtedly enhance future understandings of the etiology and management of this disorder for all.

List of Suggested Readings

Bruun, R.D., & Bruun, B. (1994). *A Mind of Its Own - Tourette's Syndrome: A Story and a Guide.* New York, NY: Oxford University Press.

Buehrens, A. (1991). *Hi, I'm Adam - A Child's Story of Tourette's Syndrome.* Duart, CA: Hope Press.

Buehrens, A., & Buehrens, C. *Adam and the Magic Marble.* Duart, CA: Hope Press.

Comings, D.E. *Tourette's syndrome and Human Behavior.* Duart, CA: Hope Press.

Handler, L. (1998). *Twitch and Shout.* New York, NY: Penguin Group.

Harris, J.C. (1995). *Developmental Neuropsychiatry - Assessment, Diagnosis, and Treatment of Developmental Disorders, Volume II.* New York, NY: Oxford University Press.

Hughes, S. (1990). *RYAN - A Mother's Story of Her Hyperactive/Tourette's Syndrome Child.* Duart, CA: Hope Press.

Hope Press
P.O. Box 188
Duart, CA 91009-0188 U.S.A.

Foundations

The Tourette's Syndrome Foundation of Canada
238 Davenport Road, Box 343
Toronto ON, Canada M5R 1J6
Tel: (416) 968-2009
Fax: (416) 964-2165

Tourette's Syndrome Association, Inc.
42-40 Bell Boulevard
Bayside, NY 11361-2820
Tel: (718) 224-2999
Fax: (718) 279-9596

References

American Psychiatric Association (APA) (1994). *Diagnostic and statistical manual of mental disorders, fourth edition*. Washington, DC: Author.

Berthier, M. L., Bayes, A., & Tolosa, E. S. (1993). Magnetic resonance imaging in patients with concurrent Tourette's disorder and Asperger's syndrome. *Journal of the American Academy of Child and Adolescent Psychiatry, 32*, 633-639.

Blakeslee, S. (1996, September 17). Studies pinpoint region of brain implicated in Tourette's syndrome. *New York Times*, p. 3.

Burd, L., Fisher, W. W., Kerbeshian, J., & Arnold, M. E. (1987). Is development of Tourette disorder a marker for improvement in patients with autism and other pervasive developmental disorders? *Journal of the American Academy of Child and Adolescent Psychiatry, 26*, 162-165.

Caine, E. D., Polinsky, R. J., Kartzinel, R., & Ebert, M.H. (1979). The trial use of clozapine for abnormal involuntary movement disorders. *American Journal of Psychiatry, 136*, 317-320.

Comings, D. E., & Comings, B. G. (1991). Clinical and genetic relationships between autism - pervasive developmental disorder and Tourette's syndrome: A study of 19 cases. *American Journal of Medical Genetics, 39*, 180-191.

Comings, D. E., Himes, J. A., & Comings, B. G. (1990). An epidemiologic study of Tourette's syndrome in a single school district. *Journal of Clinical Psychiatry, 51*, 463-469.

Como, P. (1999). *Neuropsychology: Perspectives on TS and associated disorders*. Poster session presented at the International Scientific Symposium on Tourette's syndrome, New York, NY.

Eapen, V., Robertson, M. M., Zeitlin, H., & Kurlan, R. (1997). Gilles de la Tourette's syndrome in special education schools: A United Kingdom study. *Journal of Neurology, 244*, 378-382.

Golden, G. S., & Greenhill, L. (1981). Tourette's syndrome in mentally retarded children. *Mental Retardation, 19*, 17-19.

Goldman, J. J. (1988). Tourette's syndrome in severely behavior disordered mentally retarded children. *The Psychiatric Quarterly, 59*, 73-79.

Kerbeshian, J., & Burd, L. (1986). A second visually impaired, mentally retarded male with pervasive developmental disorder, Tourette disorder and ganser's syndrome: Diagnostic classification and treatment. *International Journal of Psychiatric Medicine, 16*, 67-75.

King, R. (1999). Comorbidity in Tourette's syndrome: Pharmacological treatment in adults with a severe to profound handicap. *The NADD Bulletin, 2*, 40-44.

Kurlan, R., Whitmore, K., Irvine, C., McDermott, M. P., & Como, P. G. (1994). Tourette's syndrome in a special education population: A pilot study involving a single school district. *Neurology, 44,* 699-702.

Leckman, J. F., Price, R. A., Walkup, J. T., Ort, S., Pauls, D. L., & Cohen, D. J. (1987). Nongenetic factors in Gilles de la Tourette's syndrome. *Archives of General Psychiatry, 44,* 100.

Lees, A. J., Robertson, M., Trimble, M. R., & Murray, N. M. (1984). A clinical study of Gilles de la Tourette's syndrome in the United Kingdom. *Journal of Neurology, Neurosurgery, and Psychiatry, 47,* 1-8.

Lowe, T. L., Cohen, D. J., Detlor, J., Kremenitzer, M. W., & Shaywitz, B. A. (1982). Stimulant medications precipitate Tourette's disorder. *Journal of the American Medical Association, 247,* 1168-1169.

McDougle, C. J., Fleischmann, R. L., Epperson, C. N., Wasylink, S., Leckman, J. F., & Price, L. H. (1995). Risperidone addition in fluvoxamine-refractory obsessive-compulsive disorder: Three cases. *Journal of Clinical Psychiatry, 56,* 526-528.

Mottard, J. P., & De La Sablonniere, J. F. (1999). Olanzapine induced obsessive-compulsive disorder. *American Journal of Psychiatry, 156,* 800.

Murphy, T. K., Goodman, W. K., Fudge, M. W., Williams Jr., R. C., Ayoub, E.M., Dalal, M., et al. (1997). B lymphocyte antigen D8/17: A peripheral marker for childhood-onset obsessive-compulsive disorder and Tourette's syndrome? *American Journal of Psychiatry, 154,* 402-407.

Myers, B., & Pueschel, S. M. (1995). Tardive or atypical Tourette's disorder in a population with Down syndrome. *Research in Developmental Disabilities, 16,* 1-9.

Ozonoff, S., Strayer, D. L., McMahon, W. M., & Filloux, F. (1994). Executive function abilities in autism and Tourette's syndrome: An information processing approach. *Journal Of Child Psychology and Psychiatry and Allied Disciplines, 35,* 1015-1032.

Patil, V. J. (1992). Development of transient obsessive-compulsive symptoms during treatment with clozapine. *American Journal of Psychiatry, 149,* 272.

Perlmutter, S. J., Leitman, S. F., Garvey, M. A., Hamburger, S., Feldman, E., Leonard, H. L., et al. (1999). Therapeutic plasma exchange and intravenous immunoglobulin for obsessive-compulsive disorder and tic disorders in childhood. *Lancet, 354,* 1153-1158.

Peterson, B. S. (1996). Considerations of natural history and pathophysiology in the psychopharmacology of Tourette's syndrome. *Journal of Clinical Psychiatry, 57, (suppl. 9),* 24-34.

Peterson, B. S., & Cohen, D. J. (1998). The treatment of Tourette's syndrome: Multimodal, developmental intervention. *Journal of Clinical Psychiatry, 1998, 59, (suppl. 1),* 62-72.

Price, R. A., Kidd, K. K., Cohen, D. J., Pauls, D. L., & Leckman, J. F. (1985). A twin study of tourette's syndrome. *Archives of General Psychiatry, 42,* 815-820.

Reid, A. H. Gilles de la Tourette syndrome in mental handicap. (1984). *Journal of Mental Deficiency Research, 28,* 81-83.

Remington, G., & Adams, M. (1994). Risperidone and obsessive-compulsive symptoms. *Journal of Clinical Psychopharmacology, 14,* 358-359.

Robertson, M. M., Trimble, M. R., & Lees, A. J. (1989). Self-injurious behavior and the Gilles de la Tourette's syndrome: A clinical study and review of the literature. *Psychological Medicine, 19,* 611-625.

Serrano, C., & Pena, M. K. (1999). Efficacy of olanzapine in the management of chronic tics in a group of Puerto Rican patients. Poster session presented at the International Scientific Symposium on Tourette's syndrome, New York, NY.

Stamenkovic, M., Willinger, E., & Kasper, S. (1999). Effective treatment of Gilles de la Tourette's syndrome with olanzapine. Poster session presented at the International Scientific Symposium on Tourette's Syndrome, New York, NY.

Sverd, J. (1991) Tourette's syndrome and autistic disorder: A significant relationship. *American Journal of Medical Genetics, 39,* 173-179.

Swedo, S. E., Leonard, H. L., Mittleman, B. B., Allen, A. J., Rapoport, J. L., Dow, S. P., et al. (1997). Identification of children with autoimmune neuropsychiatric disorders associated with streptococcal infections by a marker associated with rheumatic fever. *American Journal of Psychiatry, 154,* 110-112.

Walkup, J. (1999). Epigenic and environmental risk factors. Poster session presented at the International Scientific Symposium on Tourette's Syndrome, New York, NY.

Yeates, K. O., & Bornstein, R. A. (1996). Neuropsychological correlates of learning disability subtypes in children with Tourette's syndrome. *Journal of the International Neuropsychological Society, 2,* 375-382.

Zarkowska, E., Crawley, B., & Locke, J. (1989). A behavioral intervention for Gilles de la Tourette's syndrome in a severely mentally handicapped girl. *Journal of Mental Deficiency Research, 33,* 245-253.

CHAPTER 10

Smith-Lemli-Opitz Syndrome

Małgorzata J. M. Nowaczyk & Elaine Tierney

Introduction

Smith-Lemli-Opitz Syndrome (SLOS) is an *inherited* disorder caused by a defect in the body's *synthesis of cholesterol*. It presents with a characteristic pattern of birth defects associated with mental impairment of variable degree and behavioral abnormalities. SLOS arises as a result of an inherited deficiency of an enzyme called DHCR7 that catalyzes the last step of cholesterol synthesis and causes a generalized cholesterol deficiency. The discovery of the underlying defect has led to an explosion of knowledge of this biochemical pathway. Until this discovery, there were no known biochemical disorders that caused syndromes with multiple birth defects. The gene responsible for SLOS, *DHCR7*, was identified in 1998 by three independent laboratories and specific mutations in patients with SLOS have been identified. Thus SLOS is the first *metabolic malformation syndrome* known to man with profound effects on the body plan. A number of other defects of the cholesterol synthetic pathway have been found, and a new understanding of the role cholesterol plays in human and vertebrate development and in human behavior has been reached.

Historical Note

SLOS is named after the three physicians who first described this condition: the late Dr. David W. Smith was the father of North American clinical genetics and dysmorphology; Dr. John M. Opitz is the founding editor of *American Journal of Medical Genetics*, the most widely read and quoted clinical genetics journal. They reported three unrelated boys with a distinctive facial features, microcephaly, genital anomalies, severe feeding disorder, and global developmental delay (Smith, Lemli, & Opitz, 1964). These boys were so similar in their appearance that the mother of one of them, when shown the baby picture of one of the others, was certain that it was her son's photograph. All three had an engaging personality and loved to be hugged; however, they also had difficult behaviors characterized by hyperactivity, self-injury, and autistic features. Subsequently, in his innate modesty, Dr. Opitz had suggested an alternative name derived from the first letters of the last names of the original patients, the RHS syndrome.

For the thirty years since its initial description this syndrome was one of many esoteric syndromes hidden away in dysmorphology journals and atlases, known only to clinical geneticists and dysmorphologists. However, throughout the years there were clinical clues that suggested an underlying defect of cholesterol metabolism. As early as 1963, there were reports that mouse and rat pups prevented from synthesizing cholesterol during pregnancy had birth defects similar to those observed in patients with SLOS. Patients with SLOS who died in infancy or as newborns had large adrenal glands with no lipid (specialized form of fat and cholesterol). Estriol, a pregnancy-related hormone, was suppressed in pregnancies affected with SLOS. These clinical observations have a common denominator — deficiency of the precursor of steroid hormones, cholesterol. But it was not until 1993 that two patients with SLOS had their cholesterol level measured. A special laboratory test performed at that time determined that they not only had a low plasma cholesterol, but an elevated level of another chemical as well. That compound, 7-dehydrocholesterol (7DHC), was cholesterol's immediate precursor. And so it became clear that this syndrome was caused by a simple biochemical defect in the conversion of 7DHC to cholesterol (Tint et al., 1994).

Until that time we knew of no defects of biochemical functions in the body that caused birth defects. It soon became clear that other disorders affecting cholesterol synthesis existed and that they too caused birth defects. The study of the role of cholesterol in human embryonic development constantly brings new discoveries.

Another interesting facet of SLOS is its behavioral peculiarities. Patients with SLOS have a characteristic pattern of behaviors many of which abate or improve when cholesterol therapy starts. How does cholesterol affect these changes? Is there a relationship between cholesterol and behavior, personality and psychiatric disorders? Again, evidence mounts that indeed cholesterol plays an important role in normal and abnormal behaviors. Such is the fascinating story of the discovery and the study of SLOS. See Figure 1.

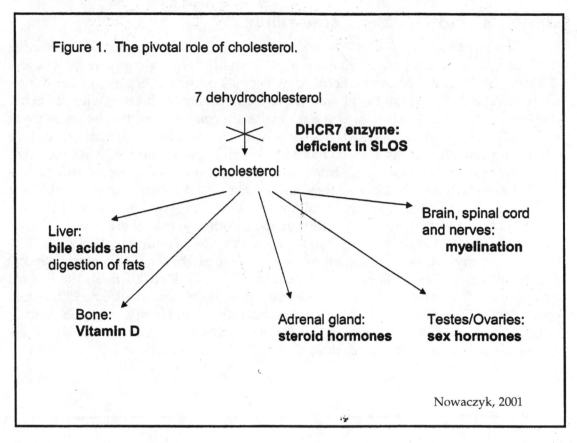

Figure 1. The pivotal role of cholesterol.

7 dehydrocholesterol

DHCR7 enzyme:
deficient in SLOS

cholesterol

Liver:
bile acids and
digestion of fats

Brain, spinal cord
and nerves:
myelination

Bone:
Vitamin D

Adrenal gland:
steroid hormones

Testes/Ovaries:
sex hormones

Nowaczyk, 2001

Biochemical Prècis

SLOS is caused by a deficiency of an enzyme involved in formation of cholesterol in the body. This enzyme, called 7-dehydrocholesterol reductase (DHCR7), converts a precursor chemical 7-dehydrocholesterol (7DHC) to cholesterol. In people with SLOS this enzyme is either absent or functions abnormally (Tint et al., 1994). As a result, there is not enough cholesterol produced in the body and 7DHC accumulates (Figure 1). Cholesterol is an important building block for the body's cell membranes, the myelination of the central nervous system, the formation of all steroid hormones (e.g., cortisol, testosterone, estrogen), and the formation of the bile acids necessary for digestion of fats. Cholesterol deficiency during prenatal life causes birth defects, while its lack in infancy and childhood causes poor growth and developmental delays. The severity of the physical findings of SLOS is related to the level of cholesterol in the plasma: *the lower the cholesterol level the more severe the condition.* Although it accumulates in the body in excessive amounts, so far there is no direct evidence that the elevated levels of 7DHC are detrimental.

Genetics and Genetic Counselling

SLOS is considered an *autosomal recessive* condition. This means that it is inherited from parents who are both carriers of an abnormally functioning gene (Nowaczyk & Waye, 2001). Only children inheriting two copies of the SLOS gene, i.e., one copy from each parent, develop the disease (Figure 2). Parents of children with SLOS are obligate *carriers*, but the presence of a normal gene compensates for the presence of the SLOS gene. This explains why parents who are completely normal can have a child with this type of hereditary condition. When a child with SLOS is conceived, she or he inherits the SLOS gene from both parents. Since both parents also carry a normal gene, any future children they might have could inherit either the SLOS or normal gene from either of them, resulting in a 25% risk of any future child inheriting two copies of the gene from their parents. In other words, there is a 1:4 chance that any child of a carrier couple would have the same condition. There is a 50% chance that any child would inherit one copy of the SLOS gene from either parents and be a carrier. Finally, there is a 25% chance that a child will inherit the normal gene from both parents and therefore not carry the SLOS gene at all. The 25% risk of occurrence is the same for each pregnancy, and does not change with the birth of normal or affected child. Therefore, *having one affected child neither increases nor decreases the risk of recurrence of the disease in the future children.*

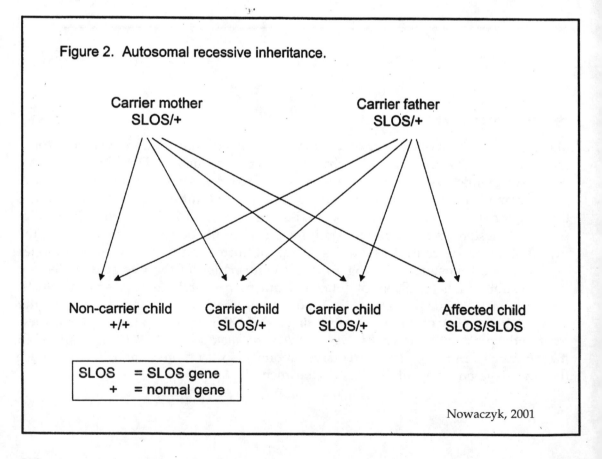

Figure 2. Autosomal recessive inheritance.

Carrier mother
SLOS/+

Carrier father
SLOS/+

Non-carrier child
+/+

Carrier child
SLOS/+

Carrier child
SLOS/+

Affected child
SLOS/SLOS

SLOS = SLOS gene
+ = normal gene

Nowaczyk, 2001

Incidence and Carrier Frequency

SLOS is most common among populations of western and central European origin, (Nowaczyk & Waye, 2001). Estimates of the incidence of SLOS vary considerably depending on the diagnostic criteria used and the population being studied. The incidence of severe SLOS in the former Czechoslovakia is estimated to be between 1 in 10,000 and 1 in 20,000, while SLOS occurs only slightly less frequently in the more mixed populations of the United Kingdom and North America. SLOS is estimated at 1 in 30,000 for New England (Holmes, 1996), 1 in 20,000 for British Columbia (Lowry & Yong, 1980), and 1 in 26,500 for Ontario (Nowaczyk, McCaughey, Whelan, & Porter, 2001). However, incidence information may be influenced by the fact that in mildly affected patients the diagnosis of SLOS may be missed. In addition, these estimates may not include the most severe cases, which result in prenatal losses or death in the newborn period.

SLOS Genetics in Numbers:	
Incidence	1 in 20,000 – 1 in 30,000
Carrier frequency	1 in 30 – 1 in 50
Risk of recurrence	1 in 4
Number of known mutations	>85
Number of SLOS genes	1

From our studies of SLOS we estimate that approximately 1:50 Caucasians in North America are carriers. In addition, by studying a large number of people who do not have relatives with SLOS we found that approximately 1 in 100 people have the most common SLOS-causing mutation called IVS8-1G→C (Nowaczyk & Waye, 2001). This mutation represents fewer than 30% of the mutations in patients with SLOS, and therefore the carrier rate for SLOS may be as high as 1 in 30 (Nowaczyk, Nakamura, Eng, Porter, & Waye, 2001).

The biochemical abnormalities of SLOS allow an accurate and rapid *prenatal diagnosis*, which is available for families *at increased risk*. SLOS can be diagnosed on material obtained either by amniocentesis at 15 to 20 weeks of pregnancy or by chorionic villus sampling, as early as 11-12 weeks of the pregnancy.

SLOS Gene – *DHCR7*, and Its Mutations

The human *DHCR7* gene was identified and mapped to the long arm of chromosome 11 in 1998 (Wassif et al, 1998; Waterham et al., 1998; Fitzy et al., 1998). Currently, more than 85 mutations have been found in SLOS patients. The most common mutation, called IVS8-1G→C, causes a complete loss of function and is found in the most severely affected patients. However, it can also be found in less affected patients if it is combined with a mutation that preserves some of the enzyme's activity. Most of the surviving patients with SLOS have at least one mild mutation, while patients with the lethal forms of SLOS often have enzymes with no residual activity. However, because there are so many different mutations, it is not possible to predict the severity of the condition accurately based on the mutations only.

Physical Features and Natural History

The physical features of SLOS present a *spectrum of variable severity* ranging from severely affected patients with lethal defects (e.g., holoprosencephaly, renal agenesis) to patients with minor physical findings who have minimal intellectual impairment or behavioral abnormalities (Kelley & Hennekam, 2000; Nowaczyk & Waye, 2001). The latter patients may be *misdiagnosed* as having idiopathic mental retardation, attention deficit-hyperactivity disorder, or autism (Nowaczyk, Whelan, & Hill, 1998). On the other extreme, patients with SLOS may have birth defects that may involve all body systems. It is the number and severity of the birth defects that determine the life expectancy and level of functioning. See Table 1.

Table 1. Birth Defects Observed in SLOS

Mouth	Cleft palate, cleft lip, excessive sublingual tissues, broad and ridged gums
Face	Epicanthal folds, narrow forehead, short nose, small chin, low set ears, forehead birthmarks, droopy eyelids
Central nervous	Small head, internal brain anomalies
Eye	Cataracts
Cardiovascular	Complex heart defects of various kinds
Gastrointestinal	Pyloric stenosis, Hirschsprung disease
Liver	Absent gallbladder
Genitourinary	Kidney cysts, absent kidneys
Genitalia	Male: hypospadias, undescended testicles, female-appearing
	Female: vaginal or uterine anomalies, hypoplastic labia
Lung	Lung cysts, other major malformations, floppy windpipe
Skeleton	Webbing of 2nd and 3rd toe, club foot, extra fingers or toes

The characteristic facial features of SLOS are microcephaly (small head size), narrow forehead, epicanthal folds, ptosis (droopy eyelids), short nose with anteverted nostrils, micrognathia (small chin), and a hemangioma (reddish birth mark) over the nasal bridge extending onto the forehead. The ears appear low-set, and are posteriorly rotated, but are otherwise normal. The classic, characteristic "SLOS face" may be very subtle in some patients (Nowaczyk et al., 1998). In cases with cleft lip or palate the facial features may be difficult to detect. Oral findings include a high-arched and narrow palate, and broad and ridged gums. *In mildly affected children the facial features may be subtle and not obvious to the untrained eye.*

Although many different forms of CNS anomalies have been reported, patients with SLOS most commonly have normal appearing brains. About 5% of patients have various forms of holoprosencephaly (a severe brain abnormality). Extra digits can be found on the hands or feet, or both. The thumb is short and placed close to the wrist, the index finger often has a subtle "zigzag" alignment. The most characteristic finding is the Y-shaped webbing of the 2nd and 3rd toes. Genital anomalies are common in the most severely affected children. The external genitalia in boys range from normal male to female appearing or ambiguous. Girls with SLOS usually have normal genitalia. Congenital heart defects are seen in about fifty percent of patients with SLOS. About one quarter of patients have kidney anomalies, such as a small kidney or its absence, kidney cysts, renal swelling, and structural abnormalities of the ureters and bladder. Laryngomalacia and tracheomalacia (floppy larynx and windpipe) may result in breathing difficulties during sleep and in sleep apnea. Abnormalities of intestinal motility (vomiting, gastroesophageal reflux, feeding intolerance, gastrointestinal irritability and allergies) as well as pyloric stenosis are frequent and contribute significantly to the morbidity. In more severely affected newborns abnormal lungs, lung hypoplasia, and Hirschsprung disease, involving variable lengths of the gut, are common. Eye abnormalities include congenital cataracts and optic nerve hypoplasia.

The *severe failure to thrive* often overshadows other problems in *surviving* children with SLOS. Newborns and infants may require tube feeding, which in many cases may be permanent. Gastroesophageal reflux with vomiting, gagging, and failure to thrive are frequent. A hypermetabolic state requiring caloric intake significantly in excess of the calculated need based on weight and level of activity is seen in many patients. Low muscle tone is universal in infancy, but it improves

Difficulties in Surviving Children
Medical problems
Failure to thrive
Feeding intolerance
Food allergies
Seizures (uncommon)
Severe photosensitivity
Sleep problems
Sleep fragmentation
Decreased sleep duration
Behavioral problems
Hypersexuality
Self injury
Autistic spectrum behaviors
Developmental delays

with age. Hypertonia, contractures, and orthopedic complications may develop in non-ambulatory children. Recurrent infections (ear infections, pneumonia) are common, as is significant photosensitivity. Other complications that may occur in patients with SLOS are adrenal insufficiency, liver disease in severely affected newborns, and difficulties with anesthesia. The type and number of medical specialists and allied health professionals involved with these patients attests to the complexity of the continuing care of even the least severely affected patients with SLOS.

Diagnosis

SLOS should be considered in **all** children presenting with *the characteristic pattern of malformations and facial features.* However, recent evidence shows that SLOS should also be ruled out in children without the severe or characteristic features but who present with *autistic-spectrum disorder, idiopathic mental retardation with/without hyperactivity, and idiopathic attention deficit disorder-hyperactivity.*

The clinical diagnosis of SLOS requires **biochemical confirmation** by demonstrating elevated serum levels of 7DHC (Tint et al., 1994). Biochemical diagnosis may also be possible on preserved samples from autopsy, neonatal screening blood spots, or stored amniotic fluid or plasma, if no blood samples are available after the death of a child. Approximately 10% of patients with SLOS have normal levels of cholesterol, and therefore measurement of **cholesterol level is not a reliable screening test** for SLOS. The levels of 7DHC can also be minimally increased in patients who are being treated with haloperidol and can lead to false positive results. In these cases the 7DHC levels are directly proportional to the dose of haloperidol, and

Medical Specialists:

Gastroenterologist

Allergist

Surgeon

Neurologist

ENT specialist

Geneticist

Infectious disease specialist

Cardiologist

Nephrologist

Urologist

Developmental specialist

Anaesthetist

Psychiatrist (for child and parents)

Health Care Professionals:
Speech therapist

Physiotherapist

Occupational therapist
Genetic counselor

Dietician

Pharmacist

Psychologist (for child and parents)

Behavioral psychologist (for child and parents)

Educational specialists

decrease to normal upon discontinuation of haloperidol.

Now that the gene for SLOS has been found, the diagnosis of SLOS can also be confirmed using molecular genetics techniques by showing that the patient inherited two copies of the SLOS gene. This method is also used for determining if other members of the family are carriers, or for verifying the diagnosis in patients on whom no samples are available. Molecular DNA testing is also available for prenatal diagnosis.

Behavioral Presentation

Many patients with SLOS who survive the newborn period often have mild to minimal physical problems; however, it is these patients that have the most severe behavioral problems because of their increased strength and ability to move.

Characteristic Behaviors of SLOS:

Sensory hypersensitivity

    tactile

    auditory

    visual

    oral tactile

Autistic spectrum behaviors

    gaze avoidance

    stereotypies

Anxiety

Self-injury

Hyperactivity/attention deficits

Backward arching

The behavioral presentation of SLOS may include *sensory hypersensitivity*, anxiety, self-injury, stereotypies (unusual movements), and sometimes aggression. Sensory hyperactivity/sensory hypersensitivity may present with intolerance of various senses such as tactile hypersensitivity and auditory hypersensitivity (Nwokoro & Mulvihill, 1997; Ryan et al., 1998). These individuals tend not to walk on grass or sand barefooted. Certain noises tend to bother them disproportionately. These are sounds that are bothersome to the general population, such as the sound of fingernails on a chalkboard, but also others. Individuals with SLOS may be bothered by sirens, bells, and vacuum cleaners; and can be bothered by any sound they hear. Oral sensitivity may also be present. The individuals tend to refuse oral feedings. This may be due to various causes including gastroesophageal reflux and possibly swallowing difficulties. When they do eat, they may be very food selective in choosing to eat few foods or choosing only foods of a certain texture. Individuals may like to smell objects as well. Visual stimulation is sometimes avoided and individuals may be overly sensitive to light or the flickering of light.

Individuals who are oversensitive to certain stimuli often are fascinated by other stimuli associated with that same sense. For example, a person who would not walk on grass or would avoid sticky items may like to rub soft and silky textures. Individuals who will not take oral feeding may place many non-edible items in their mouths and may swallow the items (pica). Individuals who dislike certain noises, such as that from a vacuum cleaner, may be fascinated by the sounds of paper being crinkled or the noise a toy makes.

Individuals often show anxiety and distress out of keeping with various situations. New social situations may be distressing, as are changes in daily routines and physical changes at home (e.g., furniture being moved).

Fifty percent of individuals with SLOS have a characteristic movement (*opisthokinesis*) in which they throw themselves backward in an arching motion that is usually very sudden in nature (Tierney et al., 2000). Thirty-five to 50% of individuals have been self-injurious at some-time (Ryan et al., 1998; Tierney et al., 2001), most commonly taking the form of biting of the forearms. The bites can leave bruises or break the skin. Chronic biting can lead to persistent skin discolouration, coarsening, and secondary infections.

> **Factors Affecting Parents/Siblings**
>
> Severe sleep deprivation
>
> Guilt ("I gave it to my child" and survivor guilt in siblings)
>
> Family planning
>
> Worry over child's future/death
>
> Safety
>
> Socialization
>
> Presence of depressive disorders
>
> Lost time from work/Financial issues

Psychiatric Risk

SLOS has been found to be associated with *autism* in 50-70% of patients. In a group of 9 subjects who started cholesterol before the age of 5.0 years, the parents were asked questions: 1) regarding the child's present state if the child was less than 5.0 years at the time of the interview, or 2) regarding the child's abilities at age 4.0 - 5.0 years if the individual was older than 5.0 years at the time of the interview. In a group of 8 subjects who started cholesterol after the age of 5.0 years, the parents were asked questions regarding the child's abilities at age 4.0 - 5.0 years prior to cholesterol being started. In this group of 8 subjects who started cholesterol after the age of 5.0 years, 88% met the autism criteria for age 4.0 - 5.0 years (Tierney et al., 2000).

Treatment

Cholesterol therapy is associated with a decrease in the number of infections, with increased weight gain and growth, with an improved sleep, and with a statistically significant decrease in autistic behaviors (Kelley & Hennekam, 2000; Tierney et al., 2000). Treatment with cholesterol has been reported to decrease irritability and hyperactivity, and to lead to a happier affect and an improved attention span (Irons, Elias, Abuelo, Tint, & Salen, 1995; Nwokoro & Mulvihill, 1997; Opitz, 1999). Self-injury also decreased with supplementation (Irons et al., 1995). Other behaviors that decreased with supplementation were aggressive behaviors (Nwokoro & Mulvihill, 1997; Ryan et al., 1998), temper outbursts, trichotillomania (compulsive hair pulling), and tactile defensiveness (Nwokoro & Mulvihill, 1997). The sensory hypersensitivity tends to decrease as individuals became older. Individuals with SLOS treated with cholesterol have also been reported to be more sociable, including initiating hugs, and more active after having had been passive (Irons et al., 1995; Ryan et al., 1998).

No side effects of cholesterol therapy have been reported to date. Although the effect of cholesterol supplementation on developmental outcome is disappointing (Kelley & Hennekam, 2000; Nowaczyk & Waye, 2001), it is possible that early administration of cholesterol therapy in infancy or in childhood may improve developmental outcomes in some patients with SLOS.

The starting dose of cholesterol is 40 to 50 mg/kg/day, increasing as needed for growth. Cholesterol is supplied either in a natural form (eggs, cream, liver) or as purified cholesterol. Because of the feeding difficulties in infants and younger children and because the diet is unpalatable, tube feeding is often required. Medical and surgical management of gastroesophageal reflux is required in many cases.

When necessary, fresh frozen plasma is used as a source of cholesterol for rapid management of infections or surgical procedures. Occasionally, when acutely ill, patients with SLOS might develop overt adrenal insufficiency requiring treatment. There is limited evidence that statins (a group of medications used to lower cholesterol in adults with abnormally high levels), may improve residual DHCR7 enzyme activity in some select patients leading to the increase in plasma cholesterol levels. Surgical treatment is required for birth defects such as congenital heart defects, Hirschsprung disease, pyloric stenosis, and skeletal anomalies.

Some of the medications that are used to treat behavioral and psychiatric disorders lower the production of cholesterol by interfering with DHCR7. But, despite the potential lowering of cholesterol production, positive benefits of the medicines may help the individual. Mildly to moderately elevated levels of 7DHC have been observed by one of us (MJMN) in three psychiatric patients without SLOS who were treated with haloperidol; 7DHC levels were directly proportional to the dose of haloperidol, and decreased to normal upon discontinuation of haloperidol therapy.

Physical Needs and Assistive Devices

Because of muscle weakness and orthopaedic abnormalities, individuals may require the assistance of physical and occupational therapists. Various devices are required to assist in mobility and strength building and to correct orthopaedic problems. These may include splints and braces for feet, standing boards, walkers, and wheelchairs or scooters for individuals more affected. Individuals who have a gastric tube will often have an automated device referred to as a "feeding pump" that delivers nutrition to the stomach via the gastric tube at the rate at which it is programmed.

Individuals with SLOS usually have difficulties in understanding spoken language as is described below. They have difficulty in understanding spoken words and engaging in reciprocal conversation (dialogue). This is referred to as receptive (understanding/hearing) and expressive (speaking) language difficulties. Because these individuals can understand so much more than they can communicate verbally, pictures can be used (as detailed below) to allow the persons to express their needs. These pictures can be placed on electronic devices and are described below under communication. Educational aids are listed below under "Education opportunities."

Psychological Features and Vulnerabilities

Skill Development and Learning

Individuals gain skills through toy use. Younger children and individuals who are more severely affected may benefit from toys that are touch- or switch-activated.

School curriculum and other programs for child development and learning should emphasize visual aids. These visual aids can be used in both school assignments and communication in the classrooms or vocational settings. An example is the use of a board on the wall that has cards that show the sequence of activities for that day. Since individuals with autism have the similar language difficulties and features that individuals with SLOS also have, children with SLOS may benefit from an autism school curriculum. It appears that for many of the individuals who take cholesterol supplementation, development and learning may increase after cholesterol supplementation begins.

Communication

Individuals with SLOS generally present with severe language impairment with greater receptive than expressive language abilities (Kelley, 1996; Nwokoro & Mulvihill, 1997; Tint et al., 1994).

Similar types of difficulties are often seen in individuals with autism and various other genetic disorders. Because of the difficulties with spoken language, pictures or photographs can be used to communicate effectively. The use of pictures in this manner has been called Functional Communication Training (FCT) and is also often referred to as the Picture Exchange Communication Training (PECT). The pictures can be attached to an object on which the child can touch the pictures. The object can be a device that plays a voice recording when touched. The individual's parent or guardian can record their voice message that says something such as "doll." Thus, when the child touches the picture of a doll, the device will state "doll" and will reinforce the child's understanding of the object and the spoken word. Devices that hold the pictures can be a round base holding 1 picture, a small board that can hold a few pictures, or boards and computers that can hold many pictures and voice recordings. For individuals that have good motor ability, pictures can be backed with Velcro™ and the individual can pick up the picture and hand them to the person who can help to obtain the object or action desired. The pictures can also be placed on a ring on a belt that allows the individual to move the pictures around to find the ones he or she wants to show someone. Alternative keyboards can be used with computers to assist communication.

Common Myths

In working with individuals with SLOS, parents and guardians have experienced fears of behavior worsening during the teen years after puberty begins. It is unclear if behaviors are worsening during puberty more than at other ages. But, the increasing size of an individual can make the individual harder to physically control.

Social Features and Vulnerabilities of Significance

Individuals with SLOS tend to have difficulties with social interactions. It appears that after cholesterol supplementation is begun, individuals seek out interaction to a greater degree. The individuals may be affectionate and seek social interaction, but still have fewer interactions than most people and have difficulties in creating and maintaining friendships. One of the changes that may be seen with adolescents and adults is the desire for romantic relationships.

Socio-Environmental Support, Assistance, Adaptations and Vulnerabilities

Because of the social difficulties the individuals display, social skills training can help them to learn the social aspects of behavior. This training can be performed through out the day including at school. For example, when it is snack-time at school, the children can take turns acting as the "host" in which they offer the snack and the roles of the "host" and the "guests" can be practiced. Prior to social events, the socially expected interactions can be rehearsed so that the individual will have better social skills and experiences to draw upon.

Education Opportunities

The receptive and expressive language difficulties experienced by individuals with SLOS need to be taken into account by school curricula. In addition to the communication difficulties, the behavioral features such as auditory hyperactivity, difficulty with change in routine, and the presence of repetitive behaviors need also be addressed. It is essential that the school provide speech and language therapy with a speech pathologist who is trained in augmentative techniques such as picture exchange as described above. Augmentative communication technology is required for most individuals and it is essential that the various means of communication are used across the day at school in all classes. Individuals usually require occupational therapy intervention to evaluate for and teach means of better hand usage. Devices such as computers and adapted pencil grips may be used. For children who ride on buses, seat-belt restraints may be required.

Adulthood and Vocational

Adults with SLOS have been reported to have profound mental retardation to normal IQ (Kelley, 1997; Lowry & Yong, 1980; Opitz, 1999). Some adults with SLOS may present with behavioral characteristics of autism spectrum disorders. It may be helpful to have the parents/guardians share information regarding SLOS and autism symptoms so that the day programs or vocational programs can better serve the individuals' needs.

Socio-Sexual

Patients with severe forms of SLOS often have delayed puberty. Cholesterol supplementation has resulted in pubertal changes in a number of older patients with the appearance of facial and body hair, body odour, and acne. There are no reports of menstrual changes upon starting cholesterol. Individuals with SLOS may have normal desires for relationships.

Summary

SLOS is a inherited genetic disorder of cholesterol production. It presents with a characteristic pattern of facial features, birth defects, mental impairment and behavior. In recent years it has been found to be a lot more common than previously thought; it might be the second most common autosomal recessive cause of mental retardation. Treatment with cholesterol improves the general health and behavior of patients with SLOS, but not the intellectual outcome. Because of the complexity of medical, emotional, behavioral and developmental problems with which these patients present and their families experience, a multidisciplinary and coordinated care is required. Resources are available and an active and dedicated parent support group exists.

Resources

SLO Advocacy and Exchange
C/o Barbara Hook
2650 Valley Forge Drive
Boothwyn, PA 19061
610-485-9664
bhook@erols.com

SLO Web site:http://members.alo.com/slo97

US National Library of Medicine: http://www4.ncbi.nlm.nih.gov/PubMed/

Recommended Reading and Resources

There are many books describing autism spectrum disorders and these can often be obtained at local libraries. There are also various websites that can supply information on topics that have been dealt with by the autism community. This includes educational programming, communication techniques including picture exchange, behavioral psychology techniques and services, and educational and medical advocacy. The following Web sites are very helpful:

The National Information Center for Children and Youth with Disabilities NICHCY's Services Include listing of state resources can be reached via the Web site: http://www.nichcy.org

Personal Responses by NICHCY to Your Specific Questions—Information specialists are available to speak with you about your area of interest or concern. Call NICHCY at **1-800-695-0285** (Voice/TTY), phones answered "live" 9:30 a.m. to 6:30 p.m. EST; voice-mail all other times or E-mail nichcy@aed.org.

NICHCY Publications—

NICHCY makes available a wide variety of publications, including fact sheets on specific disabilities, state resource sheets, parent guides, bibliographies, and our issue papers, "News Digest" and "Transition Summary." Most publications can be printed off the Internet. You may also request documents in print. Their publications are also available in alternative formats upon request.

Referrals to Other Organizations and Sources of Help—

NICHCY can put you in touch with disability organizations, parent groups, and professional associations at the state and national level (USA).
Information Searches of Their Databases and Library—
They can provide an information search to your unique needs and concerns.
Materials are also available in Spanish, on disk, and as camera-ready originals.

The Web site of the Autism Society of America has information on autism spectrum disorders, and resources including information on local chapters. http://www.autism-society.org

Another Web site that may be helpful is the Autism/ Pervasive Developmental Disorders resources network: http://www.autism-pdd.net/

In order to locate a behavioral psychologist who might be able to treat difficult behaviors: The Association for Behavior Analysis (*An International Organization*). Membership directory http://www.aba.wmich.edu/memberdirectory/index.asp

For reference, including a child's right to an education: Americans with Disabilities Act Document Center: http://janweb.icdi.wvu.edu/kinder/

Car and bus seatbelts and restraints: http://www.easywayproducts.com/schoolbus.html

Biochemical and Genetic Testing for SLOS is available in Canada though the Regional Genetic Services of Southwestern Ontario at McMaster University, Hamilton, Ontario, Canada.

Canadian Paediatric Surveillance Program
Information about the national surveillance for SLOS can be found from the
Canadian Paediatric Society at http://www.cps.ca/english/proadv/CPSP

For more information on the Canadian Paediatric Surveillance Program contact
the Program Coordinator at (613) 526-9397, ext. 239, or cpsp@cps.ca.

References

Elias, E. R., & Irons, M. (1995). Abnormal cholesterol metabolism in Smith-Lemli-Opitz syndrome. *Current Opinion in Pediatrics,7*, 710-714.

Fitzy, B.U., Witsch-Baumarter, M., Erdel, M., Lee, J.N., Paik, Y.K., Glossman, H., et al., (1998). Mutation in the r7-sterol reductase gene in patients with the Smith-Lemli-Opitz syndrome. *Proceedings of the National Academy of Science, 95*, 8181-8186.

Holmes, L.B. (1996). Prevalence of Smith-Lemli-Opitz (SLO). *American Journal of Medical Genetics, 50*, 334.

Irons, M., Elias, E. R., Abuelo, D., Tint, G. S., & Salen, G. (1995). Clinical features of the Smith-Lemli-Opitz syndrome and treatment of the cholesterol metabolic defect. *International Pediatrics, 10*, 28-32.

Kelley, R. I. (1996). Smith-Lemli-Opitz syndrome. In P. J. Vinken, & G. W. Bruyn, (Series Eds.) & H. W. Moser, (Vol. Ed.), *Handbook of neurology, neurodystrophies, and neurolipidoses* (Vol. 66, 22, pp. 581-597). Amsterdam: Elsevier Science.

Kelley, R. (1997). A new face for an old syndrome. *American Journal of Medical Genetics, 68*, 251-256.

Kelley, R., & Hennekam, R. C. H. (2000). Smith-Lemli-Opitz Syndrome. In: C. R. Scriver, A. L. Beaudet, W. S. Sly, & D. Valle (Eds.), *The metabolic and molecular basis of inherited disease* (8th ed, pp.6183-6201). New York, NY: McGraw Hill.

Lowry, R. B., & Yong, S. L. (1980). Borderline normal intelligence in the Smith-Lemli-Opitz (RSH) syndrome. *American Journal of Medical Genetics, 5*, 137-143.

Nowaczyk, M. J. M., McCaughey, D., Whelan, D. T., & Porter, F. D. (2001). Incidence of Smith-Lemli-Opitz syndrome in Ontario, Canada. *American Journal of Medical Genetics, 102*, 18-20.

Nowaczyk, M. J. M., Nakamura, L. M., Eng, B., Porter, F. D.,& Waye, J. S. (2001). Frequency and ethnic distribution of the common *DHCR7* mutation in the Smith-Lemli-Opitz syndrome. *American Journal of Medical Genetics, 102*, 383-386.

Nowaczyk, M. J. M., Whelan, D. T., & Hill R. E. (1998). Smith-Lemli-Opitz syndrome: phenotypic extreme with minimal clinical findings. *American Journal of Medical Genetics, 78*, 419-423.

Nowaczyk, M. J. M., & Waye, J. S. (2001). The Smith-Lemli-Opitz syndrome: A novel metabolic way of understanding developmental biology, embryogenesis, and dysmorphology. *Clinical Genetics, 59,* 75-386

Nwokoro, N. A., & Mulvihill, J. J. (1997). Cholesterol and bile acid replacement therapy in children and adults with Smith-Lemli-Opitz (SLO/RSH) syndrome. *American Journal of Medical Genetics, 68,* 315-321.

Opitz, J. M. (1999). RSH (so called Smith-Lemli-Opitz) syndrome. *Current Opinions in Pediatrics, 11,* 353-362.

Ryan, A. K., Bartlett, K., Clayton, P., Eaton, S., Mills, L., Donnai, D., et al. (1998). Smith-Lemli-Opitz syndrome: a variable clinical and biochemical phenotype. *Journal of Medical Genetics, 35 ,*558-565.

Smith, D. W., Lemli, L., & Opitz , J. M. (1964). A newly recognized syndrome of multiple congenital anomalies. *Journal of Pediatrics, 64,* 210-217.

Tierney, E., Nwokoro, N. A., & Kelly, R. I. (2000). Behavioral phenotype of RSH/ Smith-Lemli-Opitz syndrome. *Mental Retardation and Developmental Disabilities Research Reviews, 6 (2),*131-134.

Tierney, E., Nwokoro, N., Porter, F. D., Freund, L. S., Ghuman, J. K., & Kelly, R. I. (2001). Behavior phenotype in the RSH/ Smith-Lemli-Opitz syndrome. *American Journal of Medical Genetics, 98 (1),* 191-200.

Tint, G. S., Irons, M., Elias, E. R., Batta, A. K., Frieden, R., Chen, T. S., et al. (1994). Defective cholesterol biosynthesis associated with the Smith-Lemli-Opitz syndrome. *New England Journal of Medicine, 330,* 107-113.

Wassif, C.A., Maslen, C., Kachilele-Linjewile, S., Lin, D., Linck, L.M., Connor, W.W. et al. (1998). Mutations in the human sterol r7-reductase gene at 11q12-13 cause Smith-Lemli-Opitz syndrome. *American Journal of Human Genetics, 63,* 55-62.

Waterham, H.R., Wijburg, F.A., Hennekam, R.C.M., Vreken, P., Poll-The, B.R., Dorland, L., et al. (1998). Smith-Lemli-Opitz syndrome is caused by mutations in the 7-dehydrocholesterol reductase gene. *American Journal of Human Genetics, 63,* 329-338.

APPENDIX

Acknowledgment

*Thanks to Brenda Finucane and Terry Broda
for their input on the appendix.*

Angelman Syndrome

Formerly known as *Happy Puppet Syndrome*

Incidence: 1 in 25,000 live births

Etiology: Deletion of part of maternal copy of chromosome 15q; paternal uniparental disomy; gene mutation

How to test: Methylation Analysis followed by Cytogenetic and molecular testing, if positive

Physical Characteristics

Jerky, unsteady gait

Hypopigmentation

Characteristic facial appearance:

Long face/prominent jaw

Wide mouth

Protruding tongue

Microcephaly- small head, with flat back

Deep-set eyes

Tremors (shakiness)- often get diagnosed with ataxic cerebral palsy

Behavioral Characteristics

Happy disposition

Lack of speech

Short attention span

Frequent laughter- unprovoked smiling and laughter (unknown if mood-based)

Hyperactivity- 64-100%

Grabbing others- 100%

Frequent smiling- 96-100%

Hand flapping- 84% (excited/ when walking)

Inappropriate laughter- 77-91%

Mouthing objects- 75-100%

Sleep disorder- 57-100%

Affinity for wate, shiny objects, and musical toys

Common Medical Vulnerabilities

Seizures- 90%

Seizures become less severe with age and are the only common medical problem; appear between 1 and 3 years of age

Sleep disorders

Scoliosis

Strategies
Encourage physical activity.

To avoid contractures, keep active and mobile for as long as possible.

Wheelchair will aid in mobility

Cognitive Implications

Strengths
Receptive language higher than expressive language

Weaknesses
Severe mental delay

Developmental verbal dyspraxia

No verbal imitation/sounds/actions

Strategies
Provide alternate communication strategies (i.e., picture exchange/ picture boards)

Down Syndrome

Incidence: 1 out of every 700–1,000 live births

Etiology: Extra copy of chromosome 21

How to test: Amniocentesis, chromosome studies

Physical Characteristics

Characteristic facial appearance:

Small head with flat-looking face

Small ears and mouth

Protruding tongue

Upward slant to eyes, with epicanthal folds at inner corners

Broad neck

Short stature

Hypotonia

Increased mobility of joints

Small or undeveloped middle bone of the 5th finger

Single crease across center of palm

Brushfield spots (white spots in iris)

Lack of Moro reflex

Behavioral Characteristics

Often amiable personality, a facility for imitation

Obstinacy, keen sense of the ridiculous, and excellent memory

Alzheimer's disease

15-40% of people with Down syndrome show behavioral symptoms of Alzheimer's, usually after age 45

Depression (please see Chapter 3 for discussion)

Common Medical Vulnerabilities

Congenital heart defects- 50%

Hearing loss (ear infections)- 66-89%

Ophthalmic conditions (strabismus)- 60%

Gastrointestinal- 5%

Hypothyroidism- 50-90%

Dental (crowding, periodontitis)- 60-100%

Orthopedic (atlantoaxial subluxation)- 15%

Obesity- 50-60%

Skin conditions (dry skin, eczema)- 50%

Seizure disorder- 6-13%

Risk of seizures increases with age

Males are generally sterile

Fertility rate in females is low

Women with Down syndrome may be at an increased risk for post-menopausal health disorders, such as breast cancer, depression, and osteoporosis

Alzheimer's disease

After age 30, nearly all people with Down syndrome show the plaques and tangles characteristic of Alzheimer neuropathology, although there is not a direct correlation between plaques and tangles and the severity of Alzheimer's

Preventative strategies
Regular cardiac, hearing, vision, and thyroid exams

Neck radiography after 3 years

Preventative dental care

Weight management

Cognitive Implications

Strengths
Clear developmental trajectory

Visual memory strengths

Sequential processing intact

Can learn sequential tasks well

Weaknesses
Lower IQ scores as develop across childhood/ adolescence

Developmental rate slows throughout childhood

Average IQ is 55

Strategies
Manual signs easier to acquire- bridge to verbal language

Acquisition of communication as early as possible

Break tasks into small steps (traditional tasks analysis works well)

Inclusive setting (sociability)

Fragile X Syndrome

Incidence: 1 in 1,500 males and 1 in 2,500 females

Most common hereditary cause of intellectual disabilities in all populations

Etiology: Unusual X-linked pattern related to trinucleotide repeat expansion

How to test: Analysis

Physical Characteristics

Macrocephaly

Large ears

Long, narrow face

Macroorchidism

Low muscle tone

Hyperextensible joints

Flat feet

Soft skin

Behavioral Characteristics

Speech pattern- short bursts, repeat phrases

Imitation skills with inflection

Delayed emotional reactions

Stalling- avoidance

Overreaction to minor events

Attention deficits

Verbal vs. physical aggression

Gaze aversion (not just poor eye contact)- starts at age 2

Hyperarousal is often the root of anxiety (eye contact, overstimulation); this is demonstrated by self-injury (hand, wrist-biting); mouthing objects and clothes; hand flapping

Strategies

Be aware of anxiety triggers:

Forced eye contact

Personal space

Tactile defensiveness

Emotional tone of peers and staff

Changes in routine

Auditory stimuli

Changes in environment

Common Medical Vulnerabilities

Mitral valve prolapse- only significant medical issue

Seizures- 20%

Strabismus

Scoliosis

Sinus problems

Atlantoaxial dislocation

Cognitive Implications

Strengths

Excellent long-term memory

Verbal skills

Repertoire of acquired knowledge

Expressive and receptive vocabularies

Weaknesses

Auditory-verbal short-term memory

Visual-perceptual short-term memory

Sequential processing

Sustaining attention

Integrating information

Certain visual-spatial and perceptual organization tasks

Strategies

Teach task to another student; child with Fragile X will observe and learn task

Respond well to structure and routine

Rett's Syndrome

Incidence: Primarily in females

1 in 10,000 female births

Etiology: Mutations in the MECP2 gene on the X chromosome

How to test: Molecular analysis of the MECP2 gene

Physical Characteristics

Wide-based gait, similar to Angelman syndrome

Poor circulation- cold hands and feet

High metabolic rate

Scoliosis

Very expressive eyes

Normal head size at birth, but slowed growth between 5 months and 4 years

Hypotrophic (underdeveloped) small feet

Behavioral Characteristics

Period of regression, withdrawal (normal progress from 6 to 18 months)

Loss of acquired hand and speech skills by age 1-2 years

Onset of stereotypies- hand wringing or washing, hand mouthing

Lifelong stereotypies- often unable to use hands

Self-injury- 40-50%

Common Medical Vulnerabilities

Seizures

Hyperventilation

Central breathing dysfunction

Sleep disturbance- 70%

Scoliosis

Constipation

Strategies
Pharmacological, especially for seizures

Careful monitoring of scoliosis

Cognitive Implications

Strength
Very expressive eyes

Weaknesses
Severe to profound intellectual disability

Severe, impaired expressive and receptive language develop between 1-4 years

Strategies
Communication board

Smith-Lemli-Opitz Syndrome

Incidence: 1 in 40,000 live births

Etiology: Autosomal recessive disorder of cholesterol metabolism

How to test: 7 dehydrocholesterol analysis

Physical Characteristics

Epicanthal folds

Ptosis

Microcephaly

Small jaw

Small upturned nose

2nd and 3rd toe syndachtyly (95%)

Short thumbs

Postaxial polydactyly

Cleft palate

Hypotonia

Genital malformations from hypospadias to female genitalia in boys

Behavioral Characteristics

Feeding problems as babies

Behavioral difficulties or autistic features

Common Medical Vulnerabilities

Low blood cholesterol level

Cataracts

Cardiac defect

Liver disease

Hirschsprung's disease (absent nerves in colon)

Constipation

Hearing loss is common

Strategies

Dietary therapy, aimed at correcting cholesterol deficiency

Rectal biopsy may be useful when Hirschsprung disease is suspected

Hearing tests are important due to risk of hearing loss

Cognitive Implications

Strengths
Acquisition of good language and adaptive skills is common

Weaknesses
Intellectual disability

Expressive language disorder

Strategies
Speech therapy

Audiology

Smith-Magenis Syndrome

Incidence: 1 in 25,000

Etiology: Deletion of chromosome 17P11.2 region

How to test: FISH

Physical Characteristics

Flat mid-face

Flat head shape

Broad nasal bridge

Upper lip shaped like a "cupid's bow"

Fair hair and complexion

Missing secondary lower bicuspids

Lurching gait

"stork-like" (thin) appearance to lower legs due to peripheral neuropathy

Dry skin on hand and feet

Short in stature

Short fingers

Ear anomalies

Deep, hoarse voice

Strabismus

Nearsightedness

Behavioral Characteristics

Do not make any sounds as babies

Onychotillomania (picking at/pulling at fingernails and toenails) and polyembolokoilamania (orifice stuffing) are common. In females there may be vaginal stuffing, which may appear like an indicator of sexual abuse, but actually form of self-injury

Self-injurious behaviors- hand biting (most common); head banging (many outgrow this); skin picking

Sleep disturbances- frequent awakenings at night; deficient REM sleep; early wake-up; narcolepsy-like episodes during day; abnormal melatonin metabolism

Appreciate attention, and appears to crave one-to-one interactions and may often compete with others for attention; eager to please

Perseveration- repeatedly asking the same questions

Low impulse control- aggressive hugging, prolonged tantrums, outbursts

Do not adjust well to changes in routine

Engaging, endearing, full of personality, a sense of humor

Hugging- aggressive (rib-crushing; indiscriminate hugging of others)

Self-hugging- almost like a tic "spasmodic upper body squeezing tic thing, with facial grimacing". This is involuntary and appears when excited (less common with age)

Tactile defensiveness
(may present as stripping of clothes)

Strategies
Care providers need to be:
• Emotionally neutral in response to challenges to avoid power struggles
• Comfortable with close proximity and have a good sense of humor

Typically difficult times include transitions from activities and unexpected change; therefore, try to prepare the individual for such changes

Common Medical Vulnerabilities

Some have poor vision (extreme near-sightedness, detached retina)

Hearing impairments

Sleep abnormalities-aberrant levels of melatonin, leading to disturbed biological clock and circadian rhythm

Teeth large pulp chambers and low levels of enamel; therefore, get lots of cavities

Peripheral neuropathy (numbness/tingles in fingers and toes)

Scoliosis

Chest abnormalities (pes cavus or pes planus)

Chronic ear infections-lead to conductive hearing loss and speech problems

25% have cardiac problems

Heightened risk of hypothyroidism

Seizures

Puberty can be difficult for females;

Urinary tract anomalies

Strategies
Melotonin, in order to reverse melatonin cycle

Cognitive Implications

Strengths
Long-term memory for places, people, and things

Letter/word recognition

Simultaneous processing skills

Weaknesses
Moderate to mild range of intellectual disability

Weaknesses in sequential processing and visual short-term memory

Strategies
Calm, consistent classroom

Small class size

Reinforcers and motivators

Tourette Syndrome

Incidence: Males: 1-8 in 1,000 live births
                    Females: 0.1-4 in 1,000 live births

Etiology: UNKNOWN

How to test: See DSM-IV criteria

Physical Characteristics

No specific physical characteristics

Behavioral Characteristics

Symptoms begin between the ages of 2 and 15 years, but most people have symptoms by age 11

Hyperactivity and impulsivity are common

Complex motor and vocal tics occur in varying combinations and that wax and wane

Motor tics (simple): Abdominal tensing, arm, hand, or head jerking, echokinesis, finger movements, facial movements, rapid kicks, shoulder shrugs, bruxism.

Motor tics (complex): Adjusting clothing, arranging things, biting, body rocking, clapping, copropraxia, echopraxia, head banging, hitting, hopping/jumping/skipping, kissing, picking, sniffing/smelling, touching genitals (self or others), writing same word over and over

Vocal tics (simple): Barking, belching, blowing, chewing, coughing, grunting, screeching, shrieking, snorting, whistling

Vocal tics (complex): Coprolalia (in only 20% or so), counting rituals, echolalia, insults, laughing, mental coprolalia, partial words, stammering or stuttering, stereotyped expressions

Strategies
Perhaps tic reduction should not be the goal, rather awareness of the context in which tics are occurring as well as factors that increase impulse to tic

Suppression of tics can lead to lowered self-esteem and depression

Unrestriction/ encouragement of minor tics

Development of "Tourette's Pride" and preserving and fostering self-esteem ("It's OK to tic")

Education to clients, families, and caregivers

Expression through exercise, dance or music

Visiting places where tics are not as noticeable (i.e., baseball games)

Pharmacotherapy

Common Medical Vulnerabilities

Sleep disorders are common

No specific medical issues, although suppression of tics may lead to injury when they are finally released

Strategies
Pharmacological management with drugs such as SSRIs, adrenergic agonists, dopamine antagonists, calcium channel blockers, and atypical anti-psychotics

Cognitive Implications

Strengths
Organized way of thinking

Creativity

Weaknesses
Delays in speech development

20% prevalence of math and written language disabilities

Visual motor deficits on copying tasks

Fine motor skill deficits (i.e., poor handwriting)

Strategies
Create a quiet, separate space for test completion

Testing with modalities other than timed written examinations

Assigning tasks one by one, rather than as a sequence

22q Deletion Syndrome

Formerly known as DiGeorge syndrome, conotruncal anomaly face (CTAF) syndrome, Velocardiofacial syndrome, Shprintzen syndrome

Incidence: 1 in 4,000 live births

Etiology: Microdeletion on the long arm of chromosome 22

How to test: FISH test

Physical Characteristics

Characteristic facial appearance:

Flat affect (often hard to see)

Long, featureless philtrum

Thin upper lip

Small mouth

Prominent nasal root

Large nose with large tip

Narrow, "squinting" eyes

Small ears with thick, overfolded helixes

Oral clefts

Behavioral Characteristics

Hypernasal voice

At school age, often diagnosed with ADD, impulse control disorder, OCD, anxiety disorder

Depression (facial hypotonia)

In adolescence, 29%meet criteria for schizophrenia/ schizo-affective disorder (Pulver et al., 1994) and 64% meet criteria for bipolar spectrum disorder (Papolos et al., 1998)

Common Medical Vulnerabilities

Highly variable congenital anomaly syndrome (different organs affected)

Congenital heart defects- 80% born with cardiac defects ranging from minor to severe

- tetralogy of fallot

- interrupted aortic arch

- truncus arteriosus

- VSD

Immune deficiency

Feeding/swallowing problems

Hypocalcemia

Growth hormone deficiency

Cognitive Implications

Strengths
Verbal IQ

Verbal processing

Rote verbal learning and rote verbal memory

Initial auditory attention and simple focused attention

Auditory perception and memory

Word reading and word decoding

Weaknesses
Common cause of learning disability and intellectual disability

Non-verbal processing

Visual-spatial skills

Complex verbal memory

Facial processing and recall

Phonological processing

Deficits in language processing

Mathematics and reading comprehension

Williams Syndrome

Incidence: 1 in 20,000 live births

Etiology: Contiguous deletion of area on chromosome 7

How to test: FISH test

Physical Characteristics

Characteristic face:

Elfin-like appearance

Short, upturned nose

Long philtrum

Broad forehead with bitemporal narrowing

Full cheeks

Puffiness under the eyes

Prominent earlobes

70% have starburst pattern in iris

Hoarse voice

Hyperextensible joints

Behavioral Characteristics

Sociability

High rates of anxiety/fears/phobias

Friendly demeanor- no stranger anxiety

95%- Hyperacusis/hypersensitivity to sound-increased startle response (cover ears)

Musical talents- increased interest in music; perfect pitch

Difficulty making or keeping friends

Vulnerable to exploitation

Strategies

Music therapy or lessons

Minimize distractions (Ritalin)

Sound sensitivity management

Be attuned to obsessions- set boundaries

Social skills training

Anxiety/phobia management

Comfort/reassure/move on

Cognitive behavior therapy-systematic desensitization

Attune to underlying sadness/depression

Common Medical Vulnerabilities

Infantile hypercalcemia

Supravalvular aortic sclerosis- at least 75%

Other cardiac problems

Hypertension

Peptic ulcers, diverticulitis

Constipation, abdominal pain

Otitis Media

Premature aging of the skin

Tendency to develop hernias, urinary tract infections, and bladder diverticulae

Strabismus

Atlantoaxial dislocation

Strategies

Low calcium diet

Cardiologist

Cognitive Implications

Strengths

Verbal abilities and expressive language

Facial recognition

Musical talents

Weaknesses

Mild to moderate ID

Major impairments in visual spatial tasks

Strategies

Talk through problems-verbal mediation

Learning to read- letter/sound associations

Learning to write- raised line paper

AUTHORS

Anne S. Bassett, M.D., F.R.C.P.C.

Clinical Genetics Research Program
Centre for Addiction and Mental Health
1001 Queen Street West
Toronto, ON, Canada M6J 1H4

Anne S. Bassett is a Professor of Psychiatry at the University of Toronto and a senior psychiatric genetics researcher at the Centre for Addiction and Mental Health. Her research and clinical work focus on genetic subtypes of schizophrenia and 22q deletion syndrome.

Kerry E. Boyd M.D., F.R.C.P.C.

Area Resource Team
Hamilton Health Sciences
Chedoke Site, Residence 36
P.O. Box 2000
Hamilton, ON, Canada L8N 3Z5
Kerry Boyd is the staff psychiatrist with the Area Resource Service, Hamilton Health Sciences, an interdisciplinary team serving the dually diagnosed in Ontario.

Eva Chow, M.D., M.P.H., F.R.C.P.C.

Clinical Genetics Research Program
Centre for Addiction and Mental Health
1001 Queen Street West
Toronto, ON, Canada M6J 1H4
eva.chow@utoronto.ca

Eva Chow is a psychiatrist and researcher with the Centre for Addiction and Mental Health and the University of Toronto. She has a research interest in the neuropsychiatric phenotype of 22q11 deletion syndrome.

Garry Fay

Regional Clinical Service Co-ordinator
Developmental Disabilities Program
North Bay Psychiatric Hospital
Box 3010, Highway 11 North
North Bay, ON, Canada P1B 8L1
Garry Fay is the Clinical Service Co-ordinator for the Developmental Disabilities Program at North Bay Pschiatric Hospital. He has 19 years experience in the field of mental health and the last 6 with Developmental Disabilities.

Brenda Finucane, M.S., C.G.C.

Director, Genetic Services
Elwyn, Inc.
111 Elwyn Road
Elwyn, PA 19063
Ph. 610-891-2313
Fax: 610-891-2377

Brenda Finucane is a genetic counselor and Director of Genetic Services at Elwyn, Inc., a private, nonprofit corporation which provides services for people with developmental disabilities. She has gained national recognition for her expertise with genetic causes of mental retardation, notably fragile X and Smith-Magenis syndromes. She is widely published and has a particular interest in the practical implications of genetic diagnosis for behavioral and educational management.

Sandra Fisman, M.B., B.Ch., F.R.C.P.C.

Professor and Chair, Department of Psychiatry,
Western Faculty of Medicine and Dentistry
Chief of Psychiatry, UWO Affiliated Hospitals
London Health Sciences Centre, University Campus
339 Windermere Road
London, ON, Canada N6A 5A5
Phone: 519-663-3103
Fax: 519-663-3935
E-mail: sandra.fisman@lhsc.on.ca

Sandra Fisman is a Child and Adolescent Psychiatrist and Professor/Chair of the University of Western Ontario Department of Psychiatry in London, Ontario, Canada. She is cross-appointed in the academic university departments of Pediatrics and Family Medicine. Her qualitative research on the effects of handicapped children on other family members has been widely published. She has taught child psychiatry to pediatricians, family physicians, postgraduate trainees in psychiatry and allied health disciplines, and medical students for many years and has explored preferential methods for effectively teaching skills to practitioners and trainees.

Authors

Dorothy M. Griffiths, Ph.D.

Professor
Department of Child and Youth Studies
Brock University
St. Catharines, ON, Canada L2S 3A1

Dorothy M. Griffiths is a Professor and the Chairperson of the Child and Youth Studies Department at Brock University, St. Catharines, Ontario, and the Co-Director of the International Dual Diagnosis Certificate Programme.

Tara J. T. Kennedy, M.D., M.Ed.

Bloorview MacMillan Children's Centre
350 Rumsey Road
Toronto, ON, Canada M4G 1R8

Tara J. T. Kennedy is a Developmental Paediatrician at the Bloorview MacMillan Children's Centre. She has a Masters of Education from the Ontario Institute for Studies in Education of the University of Toronto. She is actively involved in educational projects involving physicians-in-training, practicing physicians, and the community.

Robert King, M.D., F.R.C.P.C.

North Bay Psychiatric Hospital
Highway 11 N
P.O. Box 3010
North Bay, ON, Canada P1B 8L1
Robert.King@nbph.moh.gov.on.ca.

Robert King is a consultant psychiatrist to the Developmental Disabilities Program of the North Bay Psychiatric Hospital, North Bay, Ontario, Canada.

Daune L. MacGregor, M.D., F.R.C.P.C.

555 University Avenue
Toronto, ON, Canada M5G 1X8
dmacgreg@sickkids.ca

Daune MacGregor is a Staff Neurologist in the Division of Neurology at the Hospital for Sick Children and the Clinical Director in the Department of Paediatrics at University of Toronto.

Małgorzata J.M. Nowaczyk, M.D., F.R.C.P.C., F.C.C.M.D.

Room 3N16 MUMC Campus
1200 Main Street West
Hamilton, ON, Canada
Phone: 905-521-2100, ext. 73042
Fax: 905-521-2651
nowaczyk@hhsc.ca

Małgorzata J.M. Nowaczyk is a paediatrician and geneticist and an Associate Professor of Pathology and Molecular Medicine and Paediatrics at McMaster University in Hamilton, Ontario.

Robert Pary, M.D.

Southern Illinois University School of Medicine
P.O. Box 19230
4905 Blackwolf Road
Springfield IL 62702-7857

Robert Pary is a clinical Professor of Psychiatry at Southern Illinois University School of Medicine. Dr. Pary's professional interests include teaching medical students and residents in psychiatry about persons with special needs and their mental health needs.

Dianne Pittman, M.Sc., M.D., F.R.C.P.C.

Homewood Health Centre
150 Delhi Street
Guelph, ON, Canada N1E 6K9

Dianne Pittman is a staff psychiatrist in the Community Division of the Homewood Health Centre in Guelph, Ontario, and an Assistant Clinical Professor in the Department of Psychiatry and Behavioural Neurosciences at McMaster University.

Heather Prescott, B.A. Psych

Developmental Disabilities Program
North Bay Psychiatric Hospital
Box 3010, Highway 11 North
North Bay, ON, Canada P1B 8L1

Heather Prescott is a clinician with the Developmental Disabilities Program of the North Bay Psychiatric Hospital. She has worked in the research and education field extensively, and has much experience in formatting publications, and lectures in developmental disabilities and mental health concerns.

Authors

Jay Rosenfield, M.D., M.Ed., F.R.C.P.C.

Hospital for Sick Children
555 University Avenue
Toronto, ON, Canada M5G 1X8
jay.rosenfield@sickkids.ca

Jay Rosenfield is a Project Director in the Brain and Behaviour Program at the Hospital for Sick Children Research Institute, a Developmental Paediatrician at the Child Development Centre at the Hospital for Sick Children, Co-Program Director of the Developmental Paediatrics Fellowship Program (Hospital for Sick Children and University of Toronto), Associate Professor of Paediatrics at the University of Toronto and the Director of Curriculum Design and Program Evaluation in Undergraduate Medical Education at the Faculty of Medicine, University of Toronto.

Elliott W. Simon, Ph.D.

Elwyn, Inc.
111 Elwyn Road
Elwyn, PA 19063
elliott_simon@elwyn.org

Eliott W. Simon is the Executive Director of Clinical Services for Elwyn, Inc. He has worked as a clinician, administrator and researcher in the field of developmental disabilities for over 20 years. Current interests are behavioral and cognitive developmental phenotypes of genetic mental retardation syndromes.

Jane Summers, Ph.D. C.Psych.

Residence 36, Chedoke Site
Hamilton Health Sciences
P.O. Box 2000
Hamilton, ON, Canada L8N3Z5
jsummers@hhsc.ca

Jane Summers is a Psychologist and Clinical Leader of the Area Resource Team and Behaviour Therapy Consultation Service at Chedoke Child and Family Centre, Hamilton Health Sciences. She is also part-time Assistant Professor in the Department of Psychiatry and Behavioural Neurosciences, Faculty of Health Sciences, McMaster University.

Elaine Tierney, M.D.

Director of Psychiatry
Kennedy Krieger Institute
KKI Psychiatry mail-room
3901 Greenspring Avenue
Baltimore, M.D. 21211
Office   443-923-7657
Fax   443-923-7628
Pager   410-471-8655
E-mail: Tierney@KennedyKrieger.org

Elaine Tierney is the Director of Psychiatry for the Kennedy Krieger Institute and Assistant Professor of Psychiatry at John Hopkins University School of Medicine.

Shelley L. Watson, B.A., M.Ed.

10124 87th Street
Edmonton, AB, Canada T5H 1N4

Shelley L.Watson is completing her Ph.D. at the University of Alberta in Educational Psychology, with an emphasis in Special Education. Her main interests are sexuality education, family issues, and genetic syndromes. Shelley's current research deals with family appraisal when a child is born with a genetic diagnosis.

Lonnie Zwaigenbaum, M.D., M.Sc.

Hamilton Health Sciences
Chedoke Child and Family Centre, Level 4
565 Sanitorium Road
Hamilton, ON, Canada L8N 3Z5

Lonnie Zwaigenbaum is an Assistant Professor in the Department of Paediatrics at McMaster University and Medical Director in the Hamilton Health Sciences Cleft Lip and Palate Team.